LECTURE NOT...
CARDIOLO...

LECTURE NOTES ON
CARDIOLOGY

J. S. FLEMING
M.D., M.R.C.P.(Lond. and Edin.)
Consultant Cardiologist
The United Sheffield Hospitals
and the Sheffield
Regional Hospital Board

AND

M. V. BRAIMBRIDGE
M.A., M.B., B.Chir.(Cantab.), F.R.C.S.(Eng.)
Consultant
St Thomas's Hospital
Director:
Department of Cardiothoracic Surgery

BLACKWELL SCIENTIFIC PUBLICATIONS

OXFORD   LONDON   EDINBURGH   MELBOURNE

© 1967, 1974 Blackwell Scientific Publications
Osney Mead, Oxford,
3 Nottingham Street, London W1,
9 Forrest Road, Edinburgh,
P.O. Box 9, North Balwyn, Victoria, Australia.

ISBN 0 632 08600 9

First published 1967
Second edition 1974

Printed in Great Britain by
Western Printing Services Ltd, Bristol
and bound by
Kemp Hall Bindery, Oxford.

CONTENTS

INTRODUCTION TO THE
SECOND EDITION

In the preparation of this second edition we have retained the structure and aims of the first edition. In order to present current cardiological practice, the book has been revised and several chapters rewritten. The chapter on ischaemic heart disease is now much expanded and includes modern management of arrhythmias in coronary care units and a description of the indications and techniques of saphenous vein grafts to the coronary arteries. The chapter on hypertensive heart disease has also been enlarged in consideration of the importance of this disease rather than because any major change in diagnosis or therapy has taken place over the last five years. The use of echocardiography and coronary arteriography has now become commonplace in cardiological centres and a description of the indication and value of these specialized techniques has been included. Major alterations have been necessary in the section on heart block and in the surgical treatment of congenital heart disease. Dr Webb-Peploe at St Thomas's Hospital has greatly assisted us in helping us to rewrite sections on transposition of the great arteries and single ventricle, double outlet right ventricle and Ebstein's disease.

Throughout it has been our object to present as clearly as possible the present-day management of heart disease including diagnosis, prognosis and treatment, both medical and surgical.

INTRODUCTION TO THE
FIRST EDITION

There is no lack of introductions to cardiology and little justification for another unless it is new in some respect other than the date on its cover. This book was designed as an extension of Blackwell's Lecture Notes series to provide an aid to the authors' undergraduate and post-graduate teaching, in which the students' preclinical physiological knowledge could be developed in a systematic and logical way towards the understanding of even the most complex cardiac lesions.

The main British contribution to the spectacular advances in cardiology in the last two decades has been this interpretation of each cardiac symptom and sign on a physiological basis. This advance was led by the late Dr Paul Wood and by Dr Aubrey Leatham.

The justification for placing another introduction to cardiology on the market is the commitment to this physiological approach in the presentation of cardiac disease, and also the continuation of this theme into the brief but comprehensive discussion of the surgical treatment available for each lesion.

The description of each cardiac condition is developed sequentially from its anatomy to the haemodynamic disturbances and thence to the physiological interpretation of the symptoms and physical signs. The prognosis and complications of the lesion lead rationally to description of medical treatment, indications for surgical treatment, the surgery available and its results.

It is immediately apparent that allocation of space has been heavily weighted in favour of congenital heart and acquired valve disease which lend themselves most favourably to physiological interpretation and surgical treatment. The main cardiac diseases in terms of incidence and community importance—coronary and hypertensive heart disease—are considered rather briefly, because there has been slower progress in their recognition and treatment in the last decade and because they are fully and satisfactorily covered in every textbook of medicine.

Surgical treatment also occupies a larger part of this book than most cardiological introductions. A physician has to know whether surgical treatment is possible for his cardiac patient, when it should be carried out, how his patient should be prepared for operation, what types of operation are available and what are the risks and complications of each. It is the general absence of such knowledge which has denied simple curative surgery to many patients in the last decade, and which has led to the emphasis and explanation of surgical treatment in an introduction to cardiology such as this which is designed for students who will become the general physicians and practitioners of the future.

Another function of an introduction to cardiology is the rationalization of description—aided by simple line diagrams—of the more complex cardiac lesions, which accounts for the space allotted to transposition of the great arteries, aneurysms of the thoracic aorta and others. The book has been aimed at those students who wish to widen their interest in cardiology beyond coronary and hypertensive heart disease, and the principle has therefore been adopted that almost every cardiac lesion merits inclusion, albeit briefly.

Dogmatism is inevitable in a Lecture Notes series because limited space precludes the development of conflicting theories and practice. The most widely accepted theory or practice has been outlined when alternatives exist. The results of surgery differ widely in varying centres and an attempt has been made to derive approximate mortality figures for each operation from current practice and the literature.

The pattern of description is standard throughout. The anatomy of the lesion is described, followed by its physiological disturbances. The symptoms and physical signs associated with each haemodynamic variation from normal are described. Prognosis is then outlined, followed by the types of treatment available and the benefits and risks of each. A balanced judgement on the diagnosis and treatment of any patient should then be possible.

ACKNOWLEDGEMENTS

Our indebtedness to the teaching of the late Dr Paul Wood is obvious from the text of this book. Dr Aubrey Leatham has continually stimulated our interest in the physiological background of cardiac disease, and the postgraduate teaching of Dr Graham Hayward, Dr Ronald Gibson and Dr Richard Emanuel played a large part in our understanding and knowledge of the subject. Professor Reginald Shooter gave us invaluable help in the section on bacterial endocarditis.

Some diagrams in this book are based, by kind permission, on those of other authors. That on p. 193 is modified from *Gray's Anatomy, Descriptive and Applied* (1962) 33rd edn. Longmans Green & Co.; that on p. 250 from *Grant's Method of Anatomy* (1958) 6th edn. Williams & Wilkins Co., Baltimore; and the diagram on p. 232 is modified from Hudson R.E.B. (1965) *Cardiovascular Pathology*, Edward Arnold (Publishers) Ltd.

Our grateful thanks are due to Miss Joan Dewe, Medical Artist, St Thomas's Hospital, Mrs Anne Barrett, Department of Medical Illustration, St Bartholomew's Hospital, and Mr Brandon, Photographic Department, St Thomas's Hospital, who have drawn, redrawn and photographed the diagrams. Mrs Amanda Scott and Miss Ann Gates have typed and retyped the manuscript with unfailing patience.

In the production of the second edition our grateful thanks are due to Mr J.M. Banfield, Medical Artist, St Thomas's Hospital, for drawing the new diagrams. Miss Anne Long and Mrs Rosemary Cuttler have retyped the manuscript with continual patience.

CHAPTER 1
DIAGNOSIS OF HEART DISEASE

An accurate diagnosis can usually be made from the four clinical methods of investigation of the cardiovascular system—History, Clinical Examination, Electrocardiogram and Chest Radiograph.

Special methods of investigation may be necessary to amplify the diagnosis.

HISTORY

The nature of the underlying physiological disturbances can often be ascertained from the symptoms, e.g.

Raised pulmonary venous pressure: dyspnoea, orthopnoea, nocturnal dyspnoea, cough, haemoptysis.

Inadequate coronary blood flow: angina pectoris.

Right to left intracardiac shunt: cyanosis, dyspnoea, squatting, syncopal attacks.

Congestive cardiac failure: ankle swelling, hepatic pain.

Low cardiac output: fatigue, dyspnoea.

Cardiac arrhythmias: palpitations, syncope.

Symptoms Resulting from a Raised Pulmonary Venous Pressure

Dyspnoea

DEFINITION
Dyspnoea is an uncomfortable and inappropriate awareness of respiration. Dyspnoea can result from several physiological disturbances, the most frequent cause in cardiac disease being a high pulmonary venous pressure.

MECHANISM
Any rise in pressure in the left atrium and pulmonary veins is transmitted to the pulmonary capillaries, increasing the transudation of fluid from the capillaries into the interstitial tissues of the lung. The lungs then offer more resistance to inflation and deflation and the greater muscular effort required gives the patient the sensation of

dyspnoea. Frank pulmonary oedema represents the extreme situation when severe elevation of the pulmonary venous pressure forces large amounts of fluid into the alveoli.

TYPES

Orthopnoea and Paroxysmal Nocturnal Dyspnoea describe specific forms of dyspnoea arising from a high pulmonary venous pressure. The presence of either or both is evidence that the patient's dyspnoea is caused by a high pulmonary venous pressure.

Orthopnoea

Definition   Orthopnoea means dyspnoea when lying flat which is relieved by sitting up.

Mechanism   In normal subjects the volume of blood in the lungs is increased by lying flat—right atrial filling pressure is increased and the increased filling of the right atrium and ventricle is passed on into the lungs. The pulmonary blood volume is already large in patients with a high pulmonary venous pressure and the further volume change on lying flat adds to the stiffness of the lungs.

Paroxysmal nocturnal dyspnoea

Description   Acute dyspnoea, wakening the patient from sleep, forcing him to sit upright or stand out of bed for relief. A dry cough and wheeze are commonly present during the attack, which passes off gradually after 10 to 20 minutes.

Mechanism   During the night the circulating blood volume increases in heart failure as interstitial fluid returns to the blood, and the pulmonary venous pressure may build up to high levels. The reduced awareness during sleep allows high levels to be reached before dyspnoea awakens the patient.

Acute pulmonary oedema

Description   Dyspnoea is acute and is accompanied by cough and a copious white or pink frothy sputum. There is cyanosis, perspiration, tachycardia, raised systemic blood pressure and widespread crepitations over the lungs.

Mechanism   When levels of pressure of 40 mm Hg are exceeded in the pulmonary veins the osmotic pressure of the plasma is overcome and fluid passes from the lung capillaries into the alveoli in large quantities. Rupture of pulmonary capillaries from the high pressures make the expectorated fluid pink.

GRADATION OF DYSPNOEA

Useful information about the severity of heart disease is obtained by grading the severity of dyspnoea. The following system has been found useful:

Grade 1 (Mild) Dyspnoea when undertaking unusual exertion (running, walking uphill, scrubbing).

Grade 2 (Moderate) Walking on the level causes dyspnoea.

Grade 3 (Severe) Unable to continue walking even slowly on the level. All but the lightest housework has to be given up.

Grade 4 (Gross) The slightest effort induces severe breathlessness. The patient is practically confined to bed by dyspnoea.

A history of nocturnal dyspnoea or acute pulmonary oedema places the patient in the severe grade, irrespective of the effort tolerance.

Cough

Two types of cough may be caused by a high pulmonary venous pressure:

1 Dry cough during exertion.
2 Cough productive of sputum, with wheezing.

MECHANISM

The bronchial venous return is mainly into the pulmonary veins, so that when the pulmonary venous pressure rises during exertion there is engorgement of the bronchial mucosa. This activates the cough reflex resulting in a troublesome dry cough.

Chronic elevation of the bronchial venous pressure results in an oedematous mucosa offering less resistance to infection and prone to repeated attacks of bronchitis.

Haemoptysis

As a result of the high venous pressure a bronchial vein may rupture and cause a small or large haemoptysis.

Diseases associated with a raised pulmonary venous pressure

LEFT VENTRICULAR FAILURE

The high filling pressure required for the failing left ventricle results in an increased pressure in the left atrium and the pulmonary veins.

OBSTRUCTION TO BLOOD FLOW FROM THE LUNGS

The pressure in the pulmonary veins proximal to any obstruction is high, e.g. mitral stenosis, left atrial myxoma.

Symptoms of an Inadequate Coronary Blood Flow

Angina pectoris

DESCRIPTION

Four major characteristics:

1 Quality. A crushing pain or a tight constricting sensation.
2 Site. Pain is maximal behind the sternum or across the front of the chest.
3 Radiation. Radiates into the shoulders, the neck and the jaw, down either or both arms to the fingers and through to the back of the chest.
4 Relation to exertion. Pain comes on during exertion. When exertion is discontinued the pain wears off in two or three minutes. Pain may also be provoked by anger or excitement.

MECHANISM

Insufficient supply of oxygenated blood to the myocardium results in the accumulation of metabolites which stimulate the nerve endings in the myocardium and produce pain.

Myocardial infarction

Pain is similar to that of angina pectoris in site, quality and radiation. but it is more severe and may persist for a day or two.

Causes of an inadequate coronary blood flow

1 Narrowing of the coronary arteries, e.g. atheromatous plaques in the intima, syphilitic inflammatory tissue narrowing the coronary arteries at their origin from the aorta.
2 Reduced oxygen carrying power of the blood. In severe anaemia even normal coronary arteries may be unable to carry a sufficiently large flow to meet the needs of the myocardium.
3 Increased myocardial demands for oxygen exceeding the supply, e.g. the severe ventricular hypertrophy in aortic stenosis, the very rapid heart rates in paroxysmal tachycardias.

Symptoms of Right to Left Intra-Cardiac Shunt

Central cyanosis

Blue discolouration of skin, nail beds and mucous membranes which is more marked on exertion or, in children, when crying.

Central cyanosis in congenital heart disease implies that blood low in oxygen content reaches the systemic arteries without first passing through the lungs (p. 9).

Dyspnoea

Breathlessness on exertion is present with all right to left intra-cardiac shunts. The reduced oxygen content of the arterial blood causes breathlessness by stimulating the chemoreceptors of the carotid body and the respiratory centre.

Squatting

A characteristic attitude of children who crouch on their heels when breathless, particularly after exertion.

Squatting is most commonly seen in Fallot's Tetralogy but is not specific to this condition, being occasionally seen in other forms of cyanotic congenital heart disease. By squatting the arterial oxygen saturation is improved but the precise mechanism is not known.

Syncopal attacks

Sudden attacks of loss of consciousness are common in children suffering from Fallot's Tetralogy. During the attack the child has a pallid cyanosis and profound desaturation of the arterial blood, but a normal blood pressure. These attacks occur with emotional stress, being particularly common in hospital, and may be due to spasm of the infundibulum of the right ventricle. The blood flow through the lungs is then greatly reduced, most of the blood passing across the ventricular septal defect into the aorta. Cerebral anoxia produces syncope, and if the attack is prolonged death may occur.

Symptoms of Congestive Cardiac Failure

Ankle swelling

An excess of tissue fluid follows abnormal retention of sodium and water by the kidneys in heart failure, and this tissue fluid tends to settle under the influence of gravity into the most dependent parts of the body. Thus the ambulant patient develops swelling of the feet and legs which is most marked in the evenings, whereas the patient confined to bed has a pad of oedema overlying the sacrum.

The differential diagnosis of ankle swelling includes:

1 Renal disease.
2 Deficient lymphatic drainage of the legs.
3 Deep vein thrombosis of the legs or severe varicose veins.
4 Cirrhosis of the liver.
5 Ankle swelling in normal women after standing for much of the day and most marked in the premenstrual phase when sodium and water retention is greatest.

Abdominal pain due to hepatic distension
The high systemic venous pressure of right heart failure causes hepatic enlargement and distension of the hepatic capsule. This is responsible for a dull ache in the epigastrium and the right hypochondrium. It is often aggravated by exertion which further increases the systemic venous pressure.

Symptoms of a Low Cardiac Output

Fatigue
A low cardiac output has the effect of producing a constant feeling of fatigue, presumably related to the poor blood supply to muscles and other organs. However, the complaint of tiredness is so usual in all types of illness, including psychological illness, that it cannot be regarded as reliable evidence of a low cardiac output.

Dyspnoea
The tissue anoxia of low cardiac output states is responsible for mild dyspnoea.

Symptoms of Cardiac Arrhythmia

Palpitations
Palpitation is a commonly used term for any increased awareness of the heart beat. Occasional extrasystoles are described as the heart 'seeming to miss a beat', or as the heart 'turning over in the chest'. The sudden onset of fast palpitations may represent the onset of an attack of paroxysmal tachycardia or of atrial fibrillation.

Cardiac syncope

DEFINITION
Syncope resulting from the sudden cessation of cerebral blood flow when there is an arrest of the cardiac pumping action.

DESCRIPTION
There is abrupt loss of consciousness with extreme pallor. The pupils dilate and epileptiform convulsions may occur. When efficient cardiac pumping action returns there is abrupt restoration of consciousness, accompanied by a red flush of the skin as blood flows into vessels widely dilated by the accumulation of metabolites during the brief period of circulatory arrest.

CAUSES

1 Complete heart block (Stokes Adams attack). Short episodes of cardiac arrest or of ventricular fibrillation are particularly frequent at the onset of complete heart block before the ventricular pacemaker has become well established.

2 Severe aortic stenosis. The syncope of severe aortic stenosis during exertion is a result of brief attacks of ventricular arrhythmias in some patients, induced by the exertion.

3 Paroxysmal tachycardia. Occasionally the cardiac output is so reduced at the onset of a fast arrhythmia that syncope results.

4 Left atrial ball valve thrombus, left atrial myxoma. Impaction of these structures in the mitral valve orifice is a rare cause of syncope.

CLINICAL EXAMINATION

The examination of the cardiovascular system is carried out with the patient's head and back reclining against pillows so that the thorax is at an angle of 45 degrees with the horizontal and the sternomastoid muscles are relaxed. The following features require particular attention:

General appearance. The arterial pulse and blood pressure. The jugular venous pressure and pulse. The cardiac impulses. Auscultation of the heart. The lungs. The liver. Oedema.

General Appearance

Overall build

Chronic severe heart failure may cause emaciation, and cyanotic congenital heart disease may be responsible for stunted growth and poor development. Obesity generally aggravates the effect of cardiac disease.

Anatomical abnormalities

GENETIC ABNORMALITIES

Many genetically determined disorders are easily recognized from their effects on the general body configuration. The cardiac malformations commonly associated with specific genetic defects are listed below:

Chromosome disorders

Mongolism (Triplo 21)—Endocardial cushion defects.

Turner's syndrome (XO)—Coarctation of the aorta, pulmonary stenosis.

Single gene disorders
Marfan's syndrome—aortic ectasia, dissecting aneurysm of the aorta.
Hereditary haemorrhagic telangiectasia—pulmonary arterio-venous fistulae.
Neurofibromatosis—phaeochromocytoma.
Polydactyly—common atrium, atrial septal defect.

STIGMATA INDICATING RUBELLA INFECTION
Lesions such as mental deficiency, nerve deafness and cataract in a child suggest that the mother was infected during early pregnancy by rubella. In such cases there is a strong likelihood of congenital heart disease, the common cardiac lesions produced by the virus being:
1   Patent ductus arteriosus.
2   Pulmonary valve stenosis.
3   Pulmonary artery branch stenosis.

THORACIC DEFORMITY
Great enlargement of the heart in infancy can produce a permanent deformity of the overlying chest wall with a bulging forward of the precordium to the left of the sternum.

Pulmonary hypertension complicating a left to right intra-cardiac shunt may result in an abnormally rounded configuration of the front of the chest in children.

Malar flush
Patients with a chronic low cardiac output have a dusky mauve flush of the cheeks. This colour is the result of dilated capillaries in the dermis, in which the circulation of blood is slow, and is most commonly seen in mitral stenosis complicated by pulmonary hypertension.

Cyanosis
A blue discolouration of the skin and mucous membranes caused by 5 G or more of reduced haemoglobin per 100 ml of blood in the skin capillaries.

PERIPHERAL CYANOSIS
There is a slow circulation of blood to the cyanosed part and, because the blood is in prolonged contact with the tissues, the extraction of oxygen is more complete than normal. The blood in the capillaries then has an increased proportion of reduced haemoglobin.

Vasoconstriction due to cold or as compensation for a low cardiac output is the usual cause of peripheral cyanosis, which is best seen in the lobes of the ears, the nose and the fingers.

CENTRAL CYANOSIS

Definition
Central cyanosis is defined as cyanosis caused by a reduced oxygen saturation of the systemic arterial blood.

Clinical features
The following features accompany central cyanosis and distinguish it from peripheral cyanosis:
Finger clubbing. Warm mucous membranes are blue—the tongue, lips and conjunctivae. Polycythaemia is present—abnormally high haemoglobin and haematocrit. Arterial blood, obtained by needle puncture from a peripheral artery, is desaturated—this is the absolute differentiating feature in doubtful cases.

Causes
Cardiac disease Venous blood entering the left heart without passing through the lungs i.e. right to left shunting of blood through an abnormal communication in the heart.
Pulmonary disease Inadequate oxygenation of the blood as the blood passes through the lungs.
The breathing of oxygen for a few minutes increases the oxygen tension in the alveoli of the lungs, thus compensating for poor lung function. Cyanosis due to lung disease is markedly improved, while cyanosis caused by a right to left intracardiac shunt is little affected.

DIFFERENTIAL CYANOSIS

Definition
Cyanosis more intense in the feet than in the hands when both are warm.

Cause
Differential cyanosis implies that the oxygen content of the arterial blood in the legs is lower than in the arms. Blood low in oxygen will pass from the pulmonary artery through a persistent ductus arteriosus when there is severe pulmonary hypertension. The presence of differential cyanosis is diagnostic for persistent ductus arteriosus with pulmonary hypertension.

Clubbing of the fingers

STAGES

1 Obliteration of the normal angle between the finger nail and skin on the dorsum of the finger by an increase in the soft tissues underneath the nail bed.
2 The nail becomes curved longitudinally.
3 Swelling of soft tissues of the terminal phalanges gives a drum stick appearance to the digits.

CAUSES

The exact stimulus producing finger clubbing is not known. In heart disease finger clubbing is due to cyanotic heart disease, bacterial endocarditis or left atrial myxoma.

The Arterial Pulse

The brachial arterial pulse is larger and more convenient for detailed study than the radial. For maximum information the palpating finger should compress the vessel with just sufficient force to collapse the lumen in diastole. The rise in pressure with each heart beat forcibly re-expands the wall against the finger.

The brachial pulse is analysed under four headings (Rate, Rhythm, Amplitude and Wave form).

The carotid pulse is also examined and other arterial pulses are compared with each other.

Rate

1 An abnormally fast pulse may represent:
   (i) Sinus tachycardia (sino-atrial node remains in control), e.g. excitement, fever, exertion, thyrotoxicosis, haemorrhage.
   (ii) Arrhythmia (an ectopic focus in the heart has taken over the pacemaking function from the sino-atrial node), e.g. paroxysmal atrial tachycardia, atrial flutter, atrial fibrillation, ventricular tachycardia.
2 An abnormally slow pulse may represent:
   (i) Sinus bradycardia (sino-atrial node remains in control), e.g. trained athletes, increased intra-cranial pressure, jaundice.
   (ii) Arrhythmia (a pulse rate below 40 beats per minute usually means complete heart block).

Rhythm

The normal pulse is regular apart from a slight speeding up on inspiration and slowing on expiration most obvious in youth (sinus arrhythmia). Complete irregularity indicates atrial fibrillation, but both sinus rhythm with multiple extrasystoles and atrial flutter with changing block can simulate atrial fibrillation.

EFFECT OF EXERCISE
Atrial fibrillation—the irregularity of the pulse is accentuated.
Extrasystoles—these disappear so that the pulse becomes regular.
Atrial flutter—a regular degree of A–V block becomes established, and the pulse becomes regular.

Amplitude
The amplitude of the pulse is judged by the movement of the palpating finger produced by the arrival of the pulse wave. A large amplitude pulse means that the pressure wave is large, i.e. there is a large difference between systolic and diastolic blood pressures.

LARGE AMPLITUDE PULSE

Causes
Leakage of blood from the aorta—aortic valve regurgitation, persistent ductus arteriosus, arterio-venous fistula.
Increased flow of blood from aorta through dilated arterioles—thyrotoxicosis and other high output states.
Increased left ventricular stroke volume—heart block.
Rigidity of the aorta—atherosclerosis.

Mechanism
The rapid escape of blood from the aorta in the first two groups results in a low pressure in the arterial system by the end of diastole and the large left ventricular stroke volume ejected into the aorta causes a high systolic pressure.

The very large stroke volume of complete heart block gives an abnormally large pressure peak in the aorta. A normal stroke volume produces an abnormally great pressure rise when the aorta has lost its elasticity.

SMALL AMPLITUDE PULSE

Causes
Low left ventricular stroke volume (shock, tachycardia, mitral stenosis).
Obstruction to left ventricular ejection (aortic stenosis).

Mechanism
In the low cardiac output states the volume of blood ejected into the aorta with each beat is small and the pressure rise also tends to be small.

Obstruction to left ventricular ejection reduces the speed of blood flow into the aorta during systole, thereby producing a smaller and slower than normal pressure rise in aortic stenosis.

PULSE VARYING IN AMPLITUDE

Pulsus alternans (Fig. 1.1)
Description   The amplitude of the pulse wave, in a patient in sinus rhythm, is large and small alternately.

Mechanism   Usually, in a patient in heart failure, an episode of alternans is initiated by an extrasystole. In the succeeding pause there is excessive filling of the left ventricle and the next ventricular contraction is powerful and prolonged because of the large volume to be expelled. The period available for diastolic filling of the ventricle

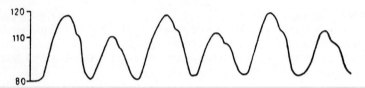

FIG. 1.1   Pulsus alternans—alternate large and small amplitude pulse

prior to the next beat is therefore short and the contraction less forceful.

Significance   Pulsus alternans is good evidence of left ventricular failure.

Pulsus paradoxus (Fig. 1.2)
Description   A marked accentuation of the normal decrease in the amplitude of the arterial pulse during normal quiet inspiration.

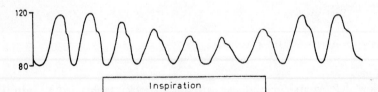

FIG. 1.2   Pulsus   paradoxus—marked   diminution   of   pulse   amplitude
during inspiration

Causes (i) Increased respiratory effort (laryngeal stridor, severe asthma).

(ii) Restriction of diastolic filling of the heart (cardiac tamponade, constrictive pericarditis).

(iii) Occasionally present in right ventricular failure.

Mechanism (i) Pulsus paradoxus in asthma.

The powerful inspiratory effort to overcome airway obstruction considerably increases the capacity of the lung vessels and thereby reduces the flow of blood out of the lungs to the left heart. The systemic arterial pulse pressure is then diminished during inspiration.

(ii) Pulsus paradoxus in tamponade.

When the diastolic volume of the heart is limited by a pericardial effusion or a rigid pericardium the normal increased filling of the right atrium and right ventricle during inspiration leaves less available volume for the left atrium and the left ventricle. Left ventricular stroke volume is reduced during inspiration and pulsus paradoxus is present.

(iii) Pulsus paradoxus in right ventricular failure.

If the failing right ventricle does not increase its output during inspiration the normal increase in the capacity of the lung vessels will restrict the flow out of the lungs into the left heart and the left entricular stroke output will decrease.

Wave form (Fig. 1.3)

The shape of the pressure wave is of diagnostic value as many abnormalities of the circulation produce characteristic changes in the form of the pulse wave which are readily detected by palpation. The normal brachial pulse has a smooth fairly sharp upstroke, a momentarily sustained peak and a quick downstroke. The dicrotic notch, representing aortic valve closure, cannot be detected clinically, but the other features are readily analysed.

Anacrotic pulse (plateau pulse, slow rising pulse)

Description The upstroke is slow with often a distinct notch on it. The time taken to reach the peak is prolonged and the entire pulse wave is of small amplitude.

Cause Aortic valve stenosis. The rate of ejection of blood into the aorta is decreased so that the duration of ejection is prolonged and the amplitude of the pulse diminished.

Water hammer pulse (collapsing pulse)

Description The upstroke is more abrupt and steep than normal. The peak is reached early, is not sustained and the downstroke is also rapid. The amplitude is usually abnormally large. The examiner's finger appreciates the sharper than normal upstroke rather than the downstroke and experiences a sharp tap with each pulse beat.

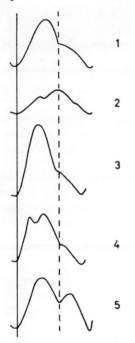

FIG. 1.3   The arterial pulse wave

1   Normal
2   Slow rising (plateau, anacrotic)
3   Abrupt rising (water hammer)
4   Bisferiens
5   Dicrotic

Causes The sharp upstroke represents the rapid ejection of blood into an empty arterial system and the rapid downstroke indicates an abnormally fast escape of blood from the arteries during diastole. A water hammer pulse is found in:

Aortic valve regurgitation   } leak at aortic level
Persistent ductus arteriosus

Systemic arteriovenous fistula   } leak at arterial level
Pregnancy

Fever, thyrotoxicosis, anaemia,   } leak due to generalized
    anoxic lung disease   arteriolar dilatation

Pulsus bisferiens

Description The upstroke is sharp to a high peak, the pressure then falls and rises again to a second peak of about the same height as the first peak before falling off. The amplitude of the pulse wave is large and the palpating finger experiences two distinct impulses with each pulse beat.

Cause This wave form indicates combined stenosis and incompetence of the aortic valve, both lesions being severe. The exact mechanism producing pulsus bisferiens is unknown.

Dicrotic pulse

Description A secondary pressure wave follows the dicrotic notch (later than the second peak of the bisferiens pulse) so that two impulses are felt with each pulse beat and may give the impression that the heart rate is twice as fast as it really is.

Cause The normal very small secondary pressure wave produced by aortic valve closure is accentuated during its transmission to the peripheral arteries when the tone of the arterial system is low— classically in typhoid fever.

Carotid pulse Carotid arterial pulsation is normally visible in the neck.

1 Invisible carotid pulsation—small pulse pressure, e.g. aortic stenosis.

2 Prominent carotid pulsation—large pulse pressure, e.g. aortic regurgitation, persistent ductus arteriosus, heart block, excitement, *or* loss of elasticity of the aorta, e.g. atheroma of the aorta, coarctation of the aorta.

Comparison of the pulses The radial pulses are compared one with the other and with the femoral pulses. The pulsations of both carotid arteries are also compared.

1 Unequal or delayed radial pulsation on one side indicates obstruction.

(i) At origin of a subclavian artery, e.g. atheromatous plaque; involvement of the origin by an aortic aneurysm; origin of a subclavian artery below a coarctation of the aorta.

(ii) Distal to origin of subclavian artery, e.g. subclavian or brachial embolus.

2 Femoral pulses small or delayed compared with radial pulses.

(i) Coarctation of the aorta (obstruction to blood flow in the thoracic aorta).

(ii) Saddle embolus.

3 Unequal carotid pulses.

Atheroma of innominate or common carotid arteries, aortic arch syndrome, dissecting aneurysm.

The Blood Pressure

The blood pressure depends primarily on the cardiac output and on the peripheral resistance, subsidiary factors being the elasticity of the aorta, the blood volume and blood viscosity.

1 The systolic blood pressure is the peak pressure achieved during the ejection of blood from the ventricle into the aorta.

2 The diastolic blood pressure varies with the peripheral resistance. If there is a rapid escape of blood from the aorta there will be a low

pressure at the end of diastole. In the absence of anatomical leaks (persistent ductus arteriosus, arteriovenous fistula) the peripheral resistance is governed by the arterioles, vasodilatation lowering the diastolic pressure.

Measurement
An inflatable cuff firmly wound round the upper arm and connected to a mercury column is used for measurement of the arterial pressure in the arm.

For accurate results the width of the sphygmomanometer cuff must be appropriate to the circumference of the arm. A cuff 5 inches in width is correct for a normal sized adult and smaller cuffs are necessary for children since a large cuff gives a falsely low reading. The systolic pressure is the highest pressure at which successive sounds are heard when auscultating over the brachial artery, and the diastolic pressure is taken at the point where the sounds abruptly become dull and muffled.

The Jugular Venous Pressure

Measurement
The patient is placed at an angle of 45 degrees with the head supported on a pillow and the pulsations of the internal jugular vein in the neck are usually clearly visible. The internal jugular vein is collapsed except for its lower part, where the pressure from the right atrium keeps it distended (Fig. 1.4). The right atrial pressure fluctuates throughout the cardiac cycle and the changing level of distension of the internal jugular vein imparts a gentle undulation to the skin of the neck which is readily distinguishable from the single sharp movement produced by carotid arterial pulsation. The vertical distance in centimetres between the top of this undulation and the sternal angle is called the jugular venous pressure and is a measurement of the pressure in the right atrium. The external jugular vein is often partially kinked and obstructed near the root of the neck and is a less reliable measure of the right atrial pressure. The jugular venous pulse is analysed for height above the sternal angle and for wave form. The normal mean pressure is 0–2 cm above the sternal angle and the wave form reveals *a* and *v* waves of approximately equal height.

Causes of a raised mean jugular venous pressure
1   High right ventricular filling pressure.
   (i) Right ventricular failure. Note from Fig. 1.5 that a failing right ventricle requires a diastolic pressure as high as 4 mm Hg to main-

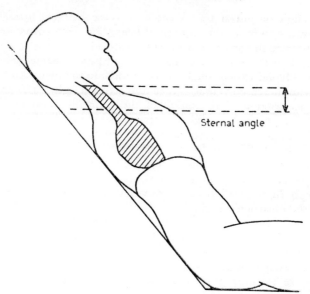

FIG. 1.4 Jugular venous pressure—vertical height above the sternal angle represents the pressure in the right atrium

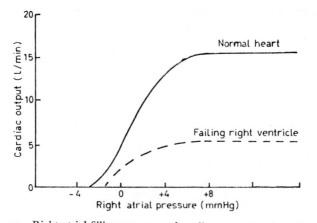

FIG. 1.5 Right atrial filling pressure and cardiac output in a hypothetical patient

tain a cardiac output of 4 litres per minute. The whole circulation adjusts to maintain a high right atrial filling pressure under these circumstances.

(ii) High output states. A slight increase in right atrial filling pressure is required even in normal hearts for the right ventricle to maintain a high cardiac output (Fig. 1.5).

(iii) Increased blood volume (overtransfusion, acute nephritis). Until the blood vessels dilate to accommodate the increased volume there is an increased venous return and a raised right atrial pressure.

(iv) Restriction of relaxation of the heart in diastole. Normal filling of the heart is impeded during diastole in tamponade and in constrictive pericarditis. An increase in ventricular diastolic pressure and in venous filling pressure is the result.

2   Obstruction to blood flow from right atrium to right ventricle (tricuspid stenosis, right atrial myxoma).

A high right atrial pressure serves to maintain the blood flow across the obstructed region.

3   Superior vena caval obstruction (involvement by bronchogenic carcinoma, or retrosternal thyroid gland enlargement).

The distended veins do not pulsate which distinguishes this cause of an elevated venous pressure.

4   Loss of negative intra-thoracic pressure (emphysema, pleural effusion, pneumothorax).

Any rise in pressure within the thorax is transmitted to the right atrium.

Abnormalities of wave form in the jugular venous pulse

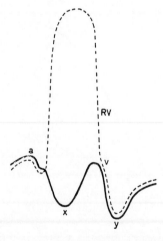

FIG. 1.6   Normal pressure waves of the jugular venous pulse—continuous line. RV (interrupted line) indicates right ventricular pressure

NORMAL

Two peaks (*a* and *v*) and two troughs (*x* and *y*) are seen during each cardiac cycle (Fig. 1.6). The waves are timed by relating them to the carotid pulse. The *a* wave precedes the carotid arterial pulse and is the pressure wave of right atrial systole. A fall in pressure follows, the *x* descent, during which the right atrium relaxes. The *v* wave is the positive pressure wave immediately after the carotid pulse and represents the rise in pressure in the right atrium as it fills with the tricuspid valve closed during ventricular systole.

At the termination of ventricular systole with the opening of the tricuspid valve, blood leaves the right atrium and its pressure falls, producing the *y* descent.

The *a* and *v* waves are of approximately equal height and do not rise more than 2 cm above the sternal angle.

ABNORMALITIES OF THE *a* WAVE

1   Large *a* wave (powerful right atrial contraction). This implies an increased resistance to blood flow from right atrium to right ventricle. The resistance may be at valve level (tricuspid stenosis, tricuspid atresia), or the right ventricle may offer more resistance to filling when its walls are hypertrophied (pulmonary stenosis, pulmonary hypertension).

2   Absent *a* wave (no co-ordinated contraction of the right atrium) i.e. atrial fibrillation.

ABNORMALITIES OF THE *v* WAVE

Large *v* waves indicate considerable reflux of blood into the right atrium during ventricular systole i.e. tricuspid incompetence.

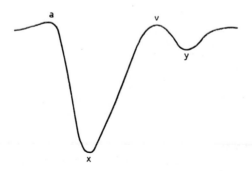

FIG. 1.7   Tamponade. Systolic descent (*x*) of the jugular venous pressure is dominant wave

ABNORMALITIES OF THE x DESCENT

Absent in atrial fibrillation (absence of atrial relaxation).

Accentuated in tamponade and in some cases of constrictive pericarditis (Fig. 1.7) (during ventricular systole blood is ejected from the heart into the pulmonary artery and into the aorta. The decrease in volume of the ventricles within the rigid pericardial box creates more volume available for filling of the right atrium from the great veins).

ABNORMALITIES OF THE y DESCENT

1 Sharp y descent. The higher the venous pressure the more abrupt is the fall in pressure when the tricuspid valve opens, provided there is no obstruction to flow from the right atrium into the right ventricle.

2 Slow y descent (Fig. 1.8). This provides evidence of obstruction

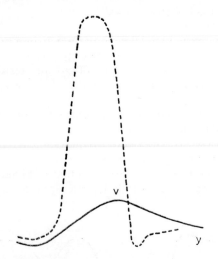

FIG. 1.8   Slow y descent of jugular venous pressure in tricuspid stenosis. Interrupted line represents right ventricular pressure

to flow from right atrium into right ventricle and is found in tricuspid stenosis or when there is tumour tissue within the right atrium.

CANNON WAVES

Large venous pressure waves synchronous with the carotid pulse, produced by atrial contraction against a closed tricuspid valve. A cannon wave therefore implies atrial contraction coinciding with ventricular systole.

Causes of cannon waves
1   Regular fast cannon waves—paroxysmal nodal tachycardia.
2   Occasional irregular cannon waves—complete heart block.
Cannon waves are only seen when atrial and ventricular systole
happen to coincide.

The Cardiac Impulses

The precordium is palpated for evidence of:
1   Cardiac enlargement.
2   Left ventricular hypertrophy.
3   Right ventricular hypertrophy.
4   Thrills.
5   Palpable heart sounds.

Cardiac enlargement

The chest X-ray gives the most reliable evidence of cardiac enlargement, but some estimate can be made from the position of the apex
beat on palpation. The point of maximum thrust is located by
placing the palm of the hand against the chest wall below the left
nipple and is accurately localized with one finger. The apex beat is
normally produced by the left ventricle and lies in the 5th intercostal space within the mid-clavicular line. An apex beat outside
these boundaries indicates cardiac enlargement if displacement of
the heart by pleural or pulmonary disease or deformity of the
thoracic cage is excluded.

Left ventricular hypertrophy

'HYPERDYNAMIC' APEX BEAT

A sustained powerful heave of the apex beat indicates a hypertrophied left ventricle, usually the result of working against the
increased pressure of systemic hypertension or aortic stenosis.

'HYPERKINETIC' APEX BEAT

An abrupt forceful apex beat of considerable amplitude is found
when the left ventricle is dilated and hypertrophied as a result of a
chronic volume overload (aortic incompetence, mitral incompetence,
ventricular septal defect).

Right ventricular hypertrophy

'HYPERDYNAMIC' RIGHT VENTRICLE

A sustained lift to the left of the lower sternum indicates a right ventricle hypertrophied as a result of working against increased pressure (pulmonary stenosis, pulmonary hypertension).

'HYPERKINETIC' RIGHT VENTRICLE

A more abrupt movement at the left sternal edge suggests right ventricular volume overload (atrial septal defect, anomalous pulmonary venous drainage).

Ventricular hypertrophy estimated by palpation must be confirmed by an electrocardiogram as occasional special circumstances can render the information obtained by palpation unreliable. A very large right ventricle may for instance form the apex beat, and systolic expansion of the left atrium in mitral incompetence can impart a thrust to the right of the sternum in the absence of right ventricular hypertrophy.

Thrills

Loud murmurs can be felt as palpable vibrations which are maximal where the murmur is loudest. Practically all cardiac murmurs may be associated with a thrill (see auscultation below).

Palpable heart sounds

The hand can appreciate the vibrations of loud heart sounds. In mitral stenosis the loud first sound is palpable at the apex, which is the explanation of the 'tapping' apex characteristic of this condition. A palpable second sound in the pulmonary area indicates a raised pulmonary arterial pressure. Gallop rhythms may be more easily appreciated by palpation than by auscultation. These sounds have considerable energy but are of low frequency not readily picked up by the ear.

Auscultation

Stethoscope

The chest piece should have a diaphragm and a bell. High frequency sounds and murmurs are heard better with the diaphragm e.g. opening snap, aortic diastolic murmur. The bell transmits low frequency sounds better, e.g. gallop sounds, mitral diastolic murmur. The bell should be applied very lightly to the chest when listening for these low frequency sounds.

Sites of auscultation (Fig. 1.9)

The site of maximum intensity of a sound or murmur is of importance in deciding its origin but complete reliance cannot be placed on this one observation, e.g. the murmur of aortic stenosis is frequently loudest at the apex. The diagnosis of the lesion responsible for a murmur is considerably more accurate when the murmur is also analysed for timing, quality, direction of selective spread and effect of respiration.

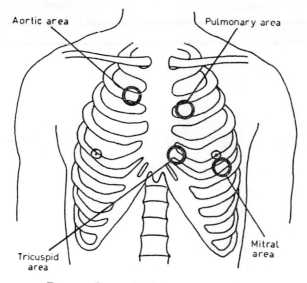

FIG. 1.9   Conventional sites of auscultation

MITRAL EVENTS

Loudest in the region of the apex beat. Best heard with the patient turned on the left side and with the breath held in expiration (heart nearest chest wall with increased flow through valve on expiration).

TRICUSPID EVENTS

Localized to the 4th left interspace at the sternal edge. Accentuated by inspiration (increased flow across valve during inspiration).

AORTIC EVENTS

Systolic murmur loud in the aortic area, at the cardiac apex and over the carotid arteries in the neck.

Regurgitant murmur loudest in 3rd and 4th left intercostal spaces at the sternal edge with the patient leaning forward in expiration (direction of the turbulent jet).

PULMONARY EVENTS

Loudest in the pulmonary area and usually localized to it. Accentuated during inspiration (low pressures in the right heart produce soft

noises which are not conducted widely, but become louder with the
increased blood flow into the lungs with inspiration).

The heart sounds
The sudden tensing of a heart valve produces vibrations both of the
valve and of any chordae tendineae and papillary muscles attached
to the valve. Many of the vibrations so produced are within the
audible range of the ear, and the normal and abnormal heart
sounds are the audible vibrations produced in this way from the four
valves of the heart.

FIRST HEART SOUND

Normal
The sudden tensing of the mitral and tricuspid valves at the onset of
ventricular systole produces the first heart sound. With the onset of
ventricular systole the left ventricular pressure rapidly exceeds the
left atrial pressure (Fig. 1.10). The mitral valve cusps are therefore

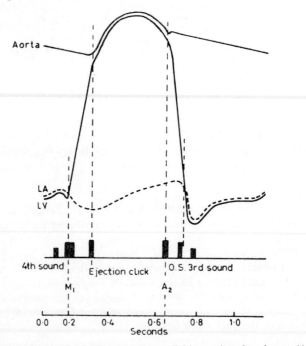

FIG. 1.10   Timing of mitral valve closure (M_1), aortic valve closure (A_2),
opening snap (O.S.), ejection click, third and fourth heart sounds in relation
to pressure changes in the aorta, the left ventricle (L.V.), and the left
atrium (L.A.)

thrust into the left atrium until suddenly arrested in apposition by the papillary muscles and chordae tendineae. The tricuspid valve is also closed by the rising pressure in the right ventricle within 20 msec of mitral valve closure, and the sounds produced by these two valves are heard as a single sound—the first heart sound (labelled M_1 in Fig. 1.10).

Loud
Mechanism At the commencement of ventricular systole the valve cusps are normally already almost in apposition as blood flowing into the ventricles has practically ceased. If the cusps are still wide apart at the onset of ventricular systole with slack chordae, an abnormally loud first sound results when they are abruptly tensed.

Causes Mitral stenosis; tricuspid stenosis; high cardiac output states (the flow of blood through the valve in late diastole remains great, keeping the cusps wide open); short PR interval (atrial contraction maintains a high flow of blood through the valve in late diastole, keeping the mitral and tricuspid valves wide apart).

Soft
Mechanism If the valve cusps are rigid and incapable of much movement, or if the cusps are already close together before the onset of ventricular systole, the first heart sound is soft.

Causes Calcification or fibrosis of the mitral valve cusps in some of the patients with mitral stenosis limit valve movement.

The valve cusps are nearly closed before the onset of ventricular systole when the PR interval is long, i.e. in 1st degree heart block.

The varying PR interval of complete heart block has the effect of altering the intensity of the first heart sound from loud, when the interval is short, to soft when the PR interval is long.

Splitting of the first heart sound
Normally the tricuspid valve closes within 0·02 sec of the mitral valve and only one sound is heard. Asynchronous contraction of the ventricles in bundle branch block, particularly right bundle branch block, may produce appreciable splitting of the first heart sound.

EJECTION CLICKS
An ejection click is a short, high frequency, clicking sound occurring shortly after the first heart sound and it arises from abnormal semilunar valves or from dilated great vessels.

Mechanism
When the ventricular pressures exceed the aortic and pulmonary

artery pressures in early systole the normal aortic and pulmonary valve cusps open widely against the vessel wall so that there is no obstruction to flow. Fusion of the cusps of these valves prevents their full opening and the abrupt arrest of the valve dome in a semi-open position produces a high pitched sound soon after the first heart sound (Fig. 1.10).

Ejection clicks can also arise from the ejection of blood into a dilated aortic root or into a dilated pulmonary artery.

Types of ejection click

Aortic ejection click, arising from an abnormal aortic valve or from a dilated aorta. This click is loudest at the apex and at the lower left sternal edge.

Pulmonary ejection click, arising from an abnormal pulmonary valve or from a dilated pulmonary artery. A pulmonary ejection click is loudest at the pulmonary area and often heard only during expiration.

Causes

Aortic click   Aortic valve stenosis, bicuspid aortic valve (a bicuspid valve cannot open completely), dilated ascending aorta, e.g. systemic hypertension.

Pulmonary click   Pulmonary valve stenosis, pulmonary hypertension (dilated main pulmonary artery).

Midsystolic Click

A high frequency clicking sound in midsystole, loudest at the apex and often followed by a late systolic murmur.

Mechanism   Redundant chordae tendineae, or papillary muscle weakness allows the mitral valve leaflets to bulge into the left atrium. The click is due to the sudden tensing of the everted valve leaflet at the time it reaches the 'end of its tether', and if the valve leaks a late systolic murmur follows.

Causes   Abnormalities of mitral valve leaflets and chordae (rupture of some chordae tendineae from whatever cause, myxomatous degeneration of mitral valve, abnormal mitral valve in Marfan's syndrome). Mitral papillary muscle dysfunction (ischaemic heart disease, including both angina pectoris and myocardial infarction).

SECOND HEART SOUND

Normal

The vibrations produced by closure of the aortic and pulmonary valves give rise to the second heart sound. The aortic valve closes at the end of left ventricular systole when the left ventricular pressure falls below the aortic pressure (Fig. 1.10) and the pulmonary valve closes at the end of right ventricular systole.

In expiration both valves close almost simultaneously and the second sound is single (Fig. 1.11). During inspiration the systemic venous return to the right ventricle is increased by the negative pressure in the thorax, right ventricular filling is increased, and right ventricular systole is prolonged. Accordingly pulmonary valve closure is delayed and the second heart sound becomes split during inspiration into an aortic component (A_2) and a pulmonary component (P_2) which follows A_2 by 0·04 sec or more.

Normal splitting of the second heart sound on inspiration is usual at all ages, but is most obvious in the young. It is best heard in the pulmonary area.

Loud second heart sound

When the sound splits on inspiration it is possible to determine which of the valve closure sounds is loud.

A_2 is loud in systemic hypertension (more forceful closure of the aortic valve).

P_2 is loud in pulmonary hypertension. P_2 is soft and not heard at the cardiac apex unless there is pulmonary hypertension.

Wide splitting of the second sound

This is heard when pulmonary valve closure is delayed either because of prolonged right ventricular systole (pulmonary stenosis) or delay in onset of right ventricular systole (right bundle branch block).

Fixed splitting of the second sound

A constant gap between A_2 and P_2 throughout all phases of respiration is the characteristic feature of an atrial septal defect. When the defect is large the right and left atria act as one common chamber and the increased return of blood to the right atrium during inspiration increases blood flow equally to both right and left ventricles. Consequently both right and left ventricular systole are prolonged and the gap between A_2 and P_2 does not alter.

Reversed splitting (Fig. 1.11)

Description In reversed splitting the second heart sound is single on inspiration and clearly split into two components during expiration.

Mechanism Reversed splitting implies that the aortic valve closes after the pulmonary valve. This occurs when left ventricular systole is prolonged or when the left ventricle contracts after the right ventricle. During inspiration pulmonary valve closure is delayed as a result of increased return of blood to the right heart, but this now has the effect of approximating pulmonary valve closure to aortic valve closure to give a single second sound.

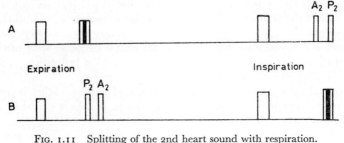

FIG. 1.11   Splitting of the 2nd heart sound with respiration.
A. Normal   B. Reversed

Causes Myocardial ischaemia or infarction (weakened left ventricle).
Aortic stenosis, coarctation of the aorta (increased resistance to ejection).
Large persistent ductus arteriosus (increase in left ventricular volume load).
Left bundle branch block (delay in activation of the left ventricle).

OPENING SNAP (Fig. 1.10)
Short, high-pitched, clicking sound closely following the second heart sound (0·60–0·12 sec), loudest medial to the apex or at the lower left sternal edge.

Mechanism
The sound is heard in mitral stenosis provided the fused valve cusps retain mobility. When the left ventricular pressure falls below the left atrial pressure the mobile valve is thrust downward into the left ventricular cavity until it suddenly tautens in its most fully open position with a high pitched snapping sound. The higher the left atrial pressure becomes the sooner will it exceed the left ventricular pressure during ventricular relaxation and the more closely will the opening snap follow A_2.

Causes
Mitral stenosis. The opening snap is absent if the valve mobility is reduced by calcification or fibrosis.

Tricuspid stenosis. A tricuspid opening snap is only occasionally present and cannot readily be distinguished from a mitral snap.

THIRD HEART SOUND (Fig. 1.10)
A low frequency, soft thud, later after the second sound, and heard at the apex (left ventricular third sound) or at the tricuspid area (right ventricular third sound).

Mechanism
During the rapid inflow phase of early diastole the left ventricle elongates, the apex moving downward and the mitral valve ring upward. This phase of rapid ventricular filling ends when the mitral valve cusps are suddenly drawn taut, stretched between the apex and the mitral valve ring, by the papillary muscles and chordae tendineae. The vibrations produced may be audible as a 3rd heart sound which occurs about 0·16 sec after A_2, at the end of the rapid ventricular filling phase. Similarly rapid filling of the right ventricle may produce a 3rd heart sound from tautening of the tricuspid valve mechanism.

Causes of a left ventricular third sound
Physiological third heart sound heard at the apex in most children and some young adults.
Left ventricular failure. The early filling phase of the ventricle is more rapid due to altered myocardial tone and the raised filling pressure.
Abnormally large flow in the filling phase (mitral incompetence, aortic incompetence, ventricular septal defect, persistent ductus arteriosus).

Causes of a right ventricular third sound
Right ventricular failure.
Constrictive pericarditis. This sound has a different mechanism and is higher pitched and earlier than the usual third sound (0·1 sec after A_2).
Sudden restriction of filling of the ventricle by the rigid pericardium plays some part in this.

FOURTH HEART SOUND (ATRIAL SOUND)
A low frequency, soft sound preceding the first heart sound.

Mechanism
This sound is heard when the left or right atrium contracts more forcefully than normal. A high atrial pressure wave reflected back

from the ventricle tenses the mitral or tricuspid valve to produce the fourth heart sound. The sound is presystolic in timing, coincides with atrial systole and is heard when a ventricle is under stress (Fig. 1.10).

Causes of a left ventricular fourth sound
Left ventricular stress—Systemic hypertension, ischaemic heart disease, aortic stenosis.

Causes of a right ventricular fourth sound
Right ventricular stress—Pulmonary hypertension, pulmonary embolism, pulmonary stenosis.

GALLOP RHYTHM
The presence of a third or fourth heart sound (or both) in addition to the usual first and second sounds is referred to as a gallop rhythm. By convention the term is used to imply a pathological condition and the physiological third sound of the young is not called a gallop.

Summation gallop. At fast heart rates an inaudible fourth sound may be superimposed on a normally inaudible third sound, the combined effect being the production of a gallop rhythm. This summation gallop disappears with slowing of the heart and does not necessarily imply ventricular stress.

Cardiac murmurs
Blood flow through the cardiac chambers is normally remarkably streamlined. Murmurs are produced when there is turbulence of the blood flow. The origin of a murmur is determined by analysing its features:
1 Timing in the cardiac cycle.
2 Site of maximal intensity and conduction.
3 Loudness and quality.
4 Influence of respiration.

TIMING IN CARDIAC CYCLE
Systolic murmurs occur during ventricular systole.
Diastolic murmurs occur in ventricular diastole.
Continuous murmurs are heard throughout the cardiac cycle.

Systolic murmurs (pansystolic, ejection, late systolic)
Pansystolic murmur   The murmur begins with the first heart sound and remains of uniform intensity throughout systole up to the second heart sound.

A pansystolic murmur is caused by a 'leaking ventricle' (mitral incompetence, tricuspid incompetence, ventricular septal defect).

Blood escapes from the ventricle as soon as it begins to contract (first sound) and continues to escape until the pressures equalize between the ventricle and atrium or other ventricle (just after second sound). Mitral incompetence is illustrated in Fig. 1.12. Left ventricular pressure exceeds left atrial pressure throughout systole from the first heart sound until after A_2, and blood escapes through the mitral valve into the left atrium giving rise to a murmur throughout systole.

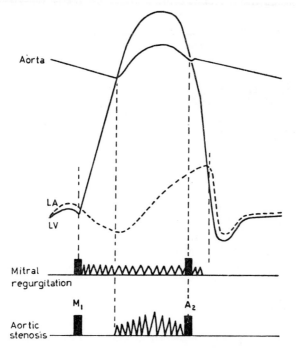

Fig. 1.12 The relationship of the murmur of mitral regurgitation and of aortic stenosis to the first and second heart sounds and to pressure changes

A pansystolic murmur is heard in the following conditions:
1 Mitral incompetence. The murmur is maximal at the apex, loudest on expiration and conducted round into the axilla.
2 Tricuspid incompetence. The murmur is maximal at the lower left sternal edge and becomes louder during inspiration.
3 Ventricular septal defect. The murmur is classically loud and rasping in quality, maximal at the lower left sternal edge and loudest on expiration.
  Ejection murmur There is a short gap between the first heart sound and the beginning of the murmur. The murmur begins softly,

reaches greatest intensity in mid-systole and ends before the second heart sound.

An ejection systolic murmur arises at the aortic or pulmonary valves when the blood flow through them is turbulent. This may be caused by narrowing of the valve orifice (aortic stenosis, pulmonary stenosis) or by a greatly increased flow through an orifice of normal size (high cardiac output states, left to right shunts). The murmur begins when the aortic or pulmonary valve opens, reaches its maximum with maximum flow in mid-systole and becomes soft again towards the end of systole. An ejection murmur must cease when flow across the valve ceases, that is, before the appropriate second sound which indicates closure of that valve. Aortic stenosis is illustrated in Fig. 1.12.

Late systolic murmur   The murmur seems to begin well after the first heart sound and thereafter increases in intensity up to the second sound. This murmur is characteristic of mild mitral regurgitation when the greatest regurgitant flow occurs in late systole. On the phonocardiogram the murmur can often be shown in fact to be pansystolic but to begin very softly.

Diastolic murmurs (early diastolic, mid-diastolic, presystolic)

Early diastolic (regurgitant)   The murmur begins immediately after the second sound and is loudest at its onset but may extend throughout diastole. High frequency and blowing in quality, the murmur is maximal usually in the third and fourth intercostal spaces close to the sternum, and may also be heard in the aortic area and at the apex.

A leaking aortic or pulmonary valve allows blood to flow back into the ventricle as soon as the valve closes (second sound), and is loudest at the beginning when the aortic or pulmonary artery pressure is highest, becoming softer as the pressure falls in diastole (Fig. 1.13).

An early diastolic murmur is heard in either aortic valve regurgitation or pulmonary valve regurgitation—usually a result of pulmonary hypertension.

The murmurs of aortic and pulmonary regurgitation are so similar that differentiation is made on other evidence, a water hammer pulse favouring aortic incompetence, and evidence of pulmonary hypertension suggesting pulmonary incompetence.

Mid-diastolic murmur   This diastolic murmur begins some time after the second heart sound. *Delayed diastolic murmur* is a more accurate description than mid-diastolic since the murmur may be short or may extend throughout the remainder of diastole. It is characteristically low pitched rumbling in character.

The murmur from a stenosed mitral or tricuspid valve begins with the resumption of flow through the valve at the end of isometric relaxation of the ventricle. The opening snap signals the end of isometric relaxation and is followed by the murmur, loudest at its onset when the atrial pressure is greatest, becoming softer as the pressure gradient between atrium and ventricle falls during diastole. This is illustrated for the murmur of mitral stenosis in Fig. 1.13. The

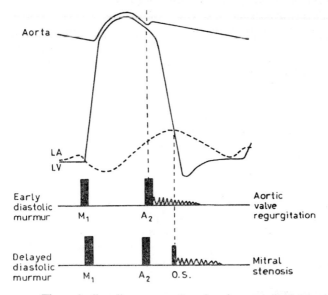

FIG. 1.13   The early diastolic murmur of aortic valve regurgitation begins immediately after A₂ (aortic valve closure). The murmur of mitral stenosis begins when the left ventricular pressure falls below the left atrial pressure, i.e. after O.S. (the opening snap)

length of the murmur is determined by the time taken for left atrial pressure to equalize with left ventricular pressure. When stenosis is severe the left atrial pressure does not fall to the left ventricular diastolic level in the time available and the diastolic murmur persists up to the first heart sound.

Causes of a mid-diastolic murmur:

1   Mitral stenosis. Murmur maximal at the apex.

2   Tricuspid stenosis. Murmur maximal at the lower left sternal edge and becoming louder during inspiration.

3   Increased blood flow across normal mitral and tricuspid valve (*flow murmurs*). Flow murmurs are low pitched, usually short and occur at the time when blood flow through the valve is rapid, that is, around mid-diastole. Mitral flow murmurs are present when there is an increased flow across that valve due to a left to right intracardiac

shunt (ventricular septal defect, persistent ductus arteriosus) or due to a generalized high cardiac output state (thyrotoxicosis, anaemia, systemic arterio-venous fistula). Tricuspid flow murmurs are usually the result of an increased flow over the tricuspid valve resulting from an atrial septal defect.

Presystolic murmur   This murmur begins in late diastole and is at its loudest just before the first heart sound (Fig. 7.2).

The presystolic murmur is the result of atrial systole forcing blood through a narrowed mitral or tricuspid valve. Atrial systole causes an increase in blood flow across the valve just before the first heart sound, provided the PR interval is normal. There is no presystolic murmur if atrial contraction is absent as in atrial fibrillation.

Causes of a presystolic murmur:
1   Mitral stenosis. Murmur maximal at the apex.
2   Tricuspid stenosis. Murmur maximal at the lower left sternal edge and louder during inspiration.

Austin Flint murmur   A presystolic murmur or a low rumbling diastolic murmur maximal at the apex and indistinguishable from the murmur of mitral stenosis.

This murmur is heard when there is free regurgitation at the aortic valve. The regurgitant stream impinges on the anterior cusp of the mitral valve and tends to hold it closed. Under these circumstances the diastolic murmurs of mitral stenosis can be produced by a normal mitral valve.

Continuous murmurs

A continuous murmur extends uninterrupted from systole into diastole and is often heard throughout all phases of the cardiac cycle.

When a communication exists between two parts of the circulation, one of which is at a higher pressure than the other throughout the cardiac cycle, blood flows continuously and a continuous murmur is produced.

Causes of a continuous murmur:
1   Escape of blood from aorta.

Persistent ductus arteriosus. Flow through the ductus is maximal towards the end of systole when aortic pressure is highest. The murmur is heard below the left clavicle and is loudest in late systole.

Pulmonary atresia. Blood flows from high pressure aortic bronchial arteries into the lungs. Again loudest in systole, often heard below the right or left clavicles or in the interscapular region at the back.

Ruptured aortic sinus of Valsalva, coronary arteriovenous fistula and any other large systemic arterio-venous fistula.
2   Blood flowing from a high to a low pressure region in the lungs.

Pulmonary artery branch stenosis.

Pulmonary arterio-venous fistula.

A *venous hum*, common in children, mimics a continuous murmur and is caused by blood flowing through the great veins in the neck and the innominate veins. It can be distinguished from the murmur of a persistent ductus arteriosus by the following features:

1 A venous hum is accentuated by inspiration whereas the murmur of a ductus is loudest on expiration.

2 Variations in posture and placing the head in different positions markedly affect the venous hum.

3 Light pressure on the neck reduces venous return from the jugular veins and may abolish the venous hum.

Pericardial friction rub

This is a superficial sound produced by the rubbing together of inflamed surfaces of the pericardium. It may be heard anywhere over the precordium and usually has two components during each cardiac cycle. It is often soft, confined to one small area and evanescent, since the rub can be abolished by a pericardial effusion separating the inflamed surfaces. The superficial quality and timing of the sound, which is confined neither to systole nor diastole, distinguishes it from a murmur.

Cause Pericarditis (p. 296).

SITE OF MAXIMAL INTENSITY AND CONDUCTION
OF THE MURMUR

This is helpful in identifying the origin of murmurs but is unreliable if used in isolation from the other features. For example aortic systolic murmurs are often loudest at the apex and aortic diastolic murmurs are loudest at the fourth left interspace close to the sternum.

(Note—A murmur is named from the lesion producing it, not from its site of maximum intensity—an aortic murmur means a murmur due to aortic valve disease and is not necessarily maximal in the aortic area.)

LOUDNESS AND QUALITY

The loudness of a murmur correlates poorly with the severity of the lesion producing it. A very loud murmur may be produced by turbulent blood flow through a small ventricular septal defect whereas the murmur is softer with larger defects. Similarly the loudness of a mitral pansystolic murmur is a poor guide to the severity of the regurgitation.

The quality or pitch of a murmur aids in its identification. High-pitched murmurs indicate a stream of blood under high pressure (aortic incompetence, mitral incompetence). Low-pitched murmurs are indicative of a turbulent blood flow under low pressure (mitral stenosis, diastolic flow murmurs).

INFLUENCE OF RESPIRATION

With inspiration the negative pressure in the thorax sucks more blood into the right atrium from the superior and inferior venæ cavæ. The blood flowing across the tricuspid and pulmonary valves is therefore increased during inspiration and increases the intensity of pulmonary and tricuspid murmurs, making this a useful clinical sign. Inspiration also brings the lung over the heart, which tends to make all sounds less well heard on the chest wall and this at times leads to confusion. In general, right-sided events are louder or unchanged on inspiration and left-sided events are louder on expiration.

Examination of the Lungs

Pleural effusions

A small pleural effusion is not uncommon in heart failure. Very large pleural effusions complicating heart disease usually indicate an underlying pulmonary infarct.

Crepitations and râles at the lung bases

The presence of excess fluid in the bronchi is indicated by inspiratory râles. Excess bronchial fluid may be the result of a high pulmonary venous pressure or due to excessive bronchial secretion caused by bronchitis. Any one of the following may be the cause of basal râles which do not therefore necessarily indicate heart failure—Chronic bronchitis, left ventricular failure, bronchiectasis, pneumonia.

Furthermore, left ventricular failure does not always cause sufficient excess of bronchial secretions to give rise to râles and crepitations, and the absence of this sign is not against the diagnosis.

Widespread fine crepitations caused by fluid in the bronchioles and alveoli are heard in pulmonary oedema.

The Liver

Enlargement

An enlarged tender liver edge below the costal margin is useful confirmatory evidence of a raised systemic venous pressure, particularly in infants when the jugular venous pressure cannot be easily determined in a short neck.

Systolic pulsation

The large systolic pressure wave of tricuspid incompetence is transmitted to the liver causing expansile systolic pulsation. This finding implies considerable tricuspid incompetence.

Oedema

The oedema fluid of cardiac failure settles under the influence of gravity into the most dependent parts of the body. Pitting oedema of the feet and ankles is therefore most often found in the ambulant patient and a pad of oedema overlying the sacrum in the patient who is confined to bed. In severe failure the oedema may be widespread and, particularly in infants, even the face can be affected.

ELECTROCARDIOGRAPHY

Preceding each mechanical contraction a wave of electrical de-polarization spreads through the heart. The depolarization begins in the sino-atrial node, situated at the junction of the superior vena cava and the right atrium, and travels over the right and left atria to reach the atrio-ventricular node. After a slight delay in the node the depolarization wave is transmitted through the atrio-ventricular bundle and its left and right branches to the Purkinje tissue of the ventricles and the ventricular muscle. A ventricular contraction follows and thereafter the ventricles are restored to their original state by a wave of repolarization.

These waves of excitation and recovery involve the movement of small electric currents within the microscopic environment of the membranes surrounding the myocardial cells. However, movements of electric currents within the heart give rise to a changing electrical field extending to the body surface. The electrocardiogram is a recording of the changing potential at the body surface caused by the movement of electric current within the heart.

Individual Components of the Electrocardiogram (Fig. 1.14)

P wave

Represents atrial depolarization. On the normal electrocardiogram it is the small initial deflection of each cardiac cycle.

Normal values: Less than 0·10 sec in duration; less than 2·5 mm in height.

QRS complex

The rapid deflections produced during depolarization of the ventricles. The upward deflection is the R wave. Any downward deflection preceding the R wave is the Q wave, and any downward deflection after the R wave is called an S wave.

Normal values: 0·09 sec or less in duration; not greater than 35 mm in total amplitude in any one lead.

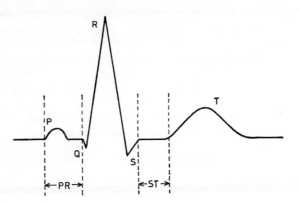

FIG. 1.14 The deflections of the electrocardiogram, P, Q, R, S and T during one cardiac cycle. PR interval measures from beginning of P to beginning of Q

ST segment
At the completion of ventricular depolarization all electrical activity within the heart ceases, and during this period the electrocardiogram shows a straight line. The ST segment begins at the termination of the S wave and continues to the onset of the T wave.

The normal ST segment is usually not more than 0·5 mm above or below the iso-electric line in any lead.

T wave
In the human heart ventricular repolarization occurs in the same sequence as depolarization. The T wave of the electrocardiogram represents ventricular repolarization and is normally positive in those leads in which the QRS complex is mainly positive.

U wave
A small deflection following the T wave, not always present, and usually of little clinical significance.

Recording the Electrocardiogram
Leads
In clinical practice the electrocardiogram is recorded twelve times in

each patient, using twelve different electrode positions. All leads record the same electrical activity of the heart but, since they are seeing it from different positions on the body surface, the deflections are different in appearance in the various leads.

BIPOLAR LEADS

These leads measure the potential difference between two points on the body surface.

Standard lead I—one electrode on the right arm, the other on the left arm.

Standard lead II—one electrode on the right arm, the other on the left leg.

Standard lead III—one electrode on the left arm, the other on the left leg.

Most modern electrocardiographs require an electrode to be placed on the right leg also, in order to obtain a more stable recording.

UNIPOLAR LEADS (SYNONYM: V LEADS)

With these leads the changing body surface potential is measured at one electrode only, the other electrocardiographic terminal being kept at zero potential.

Limb leads

aVr—one electrode on the right arm, the other at zero potential.
aVl—one electrode on the left arm, the other at zero potential.
aVf—one electrode on the left leg, the other at zero potential.

(Note—*a* preceding the unipolar leads means that additional amplification has been carried out on these leads and is short for *augmented.*)

Precordial leads

V1 to V6—one electrode is placed on the precordium in the position shown on the diagram (Fig. 1.15), while the other electrode is kept at zero potential.

Timing of the electrocardiographic events

The electrocardiogram is recorded on paper running at a speed of 25 mm per sec, each millimetre on the paper representing 1/25th (0·04) sec, and the heavier lines marked on the paper every 5 mm represent 0·2 sec. The sensitivity of the machine is set so that 1 mV of potential difference between the exploring electrodes produces a 10 mm vertical deflection on the paper.

The heart rate is found by counting the number of QRS complexes

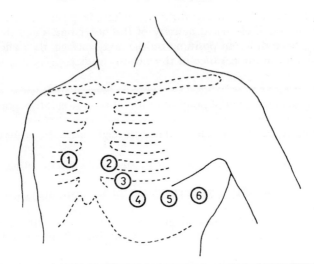

FIG. 1.15   Precordial lead positions (V leads). 1 is at 4th right intercostal
space at the sternal edge

in 3 sec (15 large squares) and multiplying by 20, or by dividing 300
by the number of large squares between two consecutive R waves.

The PR interval represents the sum of the time taken for atrial
depolarization plus the delay of the excitation process in the A–V
node and is measured from the beginning of the P wave to the
beginning of the QRS complex.

Normal value: Not more than 0·22 sec.

The Normal QRS Complex

Distinction between frontal and horizontal plane leads
The electrical forces in the heart act in three dimensions but the
standard leads record only the frontal plane components of these
forces. The precordial leads record forces from the heart directed in
an anterior or posterior direction. The standard leads are therefore
frontal plane leads and the precordial leads are horizontal plane
leads.

Standard leads (frontal plane leads)
The standard leads can be represented as straight lines connecting
the right arm, the left arm and the left leg (Fig. 1.16). Consider an
electrical force in the heart whose magnitude and direction is represented by the arrow. This force is parallel to lead I and lead I sees

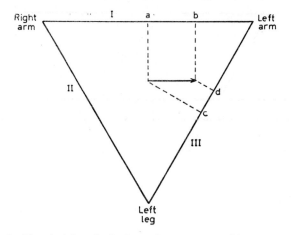

FIG. 1.16 Electrical force in the heart, large arrow, and its components in lead I and lead III

the force as if it were a force of magnitude and direction *ab*. A positive deflection is recorded by lead I, since forces travelling towards the left arm are recorded as upward deflections when lead I is used. However when lead III is used, the same electrical force has a parallel component *cd* to that lead and this is recorded as a negative deflection, since forces travelling away from the left leg are recorded as negative forces when lead III is used. Thus, although all the electrocardiographic leads record the same electrical activity of the heart, they are seeing it from different positions on the body surface, and the deflections are different in appearance in the various leads.

At any moment during ventricular depolarization there are many different electrical forces, but the average direction and magnitude of these electrical forces during this moment can be represented by a single arrow, the resultant of all these small forces. The arrows in Fig. 1.17 represent the average direction of the electrical force at various moments during ventricular depolarization. Arrow 1 represents depolarization of the interventricular septum, the first part of the ventricles to be depolarized. This force produces a negative deflection in lead I since its horizontal component is travelling towards the right arm. Similarly the force during the next part of depolarization, arrow 2, continues the negative deflection. Arrow 3 is at right angles to lead I and because this force cannot be recorded by lead I the tracing returns to the iso-electric line. Arrows 4, 5, 6 and 7 all have components running towards the left arm and are recorded as positive deflections in lead I.

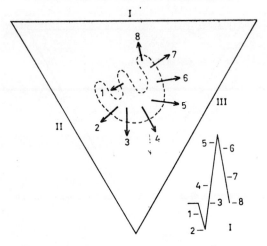

FIG. 1.17 The moment by moment movements of currents within the heart. Each arrow represents the average direction of all currents moving in the heart at one particular moment during ventricular depolarization. Eight moments during depolarization are depicted

Precordial leads (horizontal plane leads)

Leads V1 to V6 are used to pick up the forces from the heart directed in an anterior or posterior direction—an upward deflection in V1 and V2 represents an electrical force directed anteriorly and an S wave in these leads indicates that the electrical force is travelling posteriorly during the inscription of the wave.

The Mean Frontal QRS Axis

Description

When the average of all the forces acting throughout the inscription of the QRS complex is taken, the direction of this force is called the mean QRS axis.

In Fig. 1.17 the arrows represent the moment to moment direction of the electrical forces during ventricular depolarization. If the average of all these forces is taken and represented by a single arrow, the direction of the arrow is the mean (or average) direction of ventricular depolarization and is called the mean QRS axis (Fig. 1.18).

Determination

One standard lead can usually be found in which the area of the QRS above the iso-electric line is equal, or nearly so, to the area below the iso-electric line. This means that the average direction of

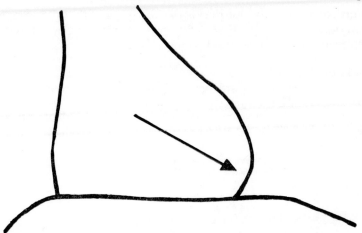

Fig. 1.18 Mean Frontal QRS Axis. Average direction of travel of the electrical forces through the ventricles during inscription of the QRS complex is represented by the arrow. This arrow is the mean QRS axis

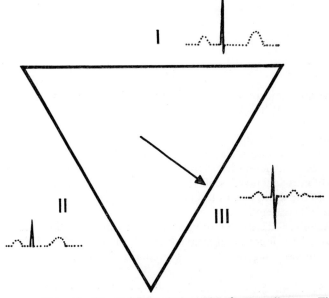

Fig. 1.19 Determination of QRS axis from the electrocardiogram. The areas of the QRS complex above and below the iso-electric line are equal in lead III. A line is drawn at right angles to lead III. The arrow head, indicating the direction of this line, is inserted by looking at the QRS complex in lead I. Lead I has a positive deflection, indicating that the direction is towards the left arm

ventricular depolarization during the inscription of the QRS complex
is at right angles to that lead. A line drawn at right angles to this lead
represents the mean frontal QRS axis (Fig. 1.19).

Axis deviation

The axis of the electrocardiogram is described in degrees according
to Fig. 1.20. The normal axis in adults lies between −30 deg and
+90 deg. An electrical axis greater than +90 deg is called right axis
deviation and left axis deviation refers to an axis less than −30 deg.

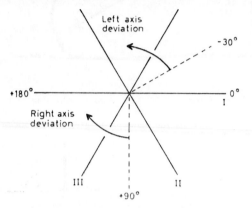

FIG. 1.20   Frontal plane mean QRS axis

Some conditions associated with axis deviation

1   Congenital heart disease
Tricuspid atresia
Ostium primum atrial septal defect } left axis deviation
Ostium secundum atrial septal defect—right axis deviation.
2   Right ventricular hypertrophy. When considerable, the increased
mass of muscle tends to shift the average direction of the depolarizing
force to the right, e.g. pulmonary stenosis; plumonary hypertension;
Fallot's Tetralogy.
3   Acquired disease of the myocardium altering the direction of
spread of the depolarizing wave through the ventricles e.g. ischaemic
heart disease; degeneration of the conducting system.

Abnormalities of the Electrocardiogram in Disease

Left ventricular hypertrophy

CRITERIA (Fig. 1.21)
1   Increased amplitude of the QRS deflection.

2   Inverted T waves in left precordial leads (V4, V5 and V6).
3   ST depression in the leads with inverted T waves.

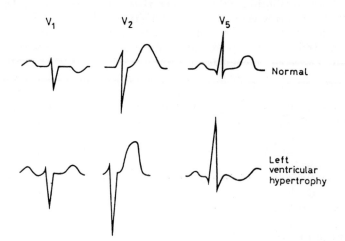

FIG. 1.21   The precordial leads in left ventricular hypertrophy

MECHANISM

1   Depolarization of the increased ventricular mass of muscle produces larger electrical forces, and the changes in potential are therefore greater than normal in the leads which best record these forces
(usually V5 and V6).

No reliable voltage criteria for left ventricular hypertrophy can be
given, but in an adult of normal build a QRS complex in any lead
greater than 35 mm in total amplitude usually indicates left
ventricular hypertrophy. Similarly a sum of S wave in V1 plus R
wave in V5, greater than 40 mm indicates left ventricular hypertrophy.

2, 3   Severe hypertrophy disturbs ventricular repolarization, possibly because of the increased tension developed in the muscle during
systole. This disturbance in repolarization is shown by inverted T
waves in leads V4, V5 and V6 and by ST segment depression in these
leads.

Right ventricular hypertrophy

CRITERIA

1   Right axis deviation of the mean frontal QRS axis.
2   Tall R waves in V1 and V2 or an RSR' pattern in those leads.
3   Inverted T waves in V1, V2 and V3.

MECHANISM

1   The contribution of the right ventricle to the total electrical forces developed during ventricular depolarization is increased when there is an increased right ventricular muscle mass. The average direction of the ventricular depolarization force is therefore shifted to the right. The axis is recognizably abnormal only when it has shifted to more than +90 deg, so that many patients may have right ventricular hypertrophy which is not detectable by electrocardiography.

2   The greater electrical forces developed in the hypertrophied right ventricle produce greater deflections in the leads recording anteriorly directed forces best i.e. V1 and V2. Therefore the R wave in V1 becomes larger than the S wave in this lead, or a second anterior wave is seen (R').

3   Repolarization of the right ventricle is disturbed because of the increased right ventricular wall tension and T waves become inverted in V1, V2 and V3.

Bundle branch block

ANATOMY OF VENTRICULAR CONDUCTING TISSUE

From the atrio-ventricular node situated in the right atrium immediately above the opening of the coronary sinus the specialized conducting tissue of the heart runs down the interventricular septum, first as a single tract (bundle of His), and then dividing into a right bundle supplying the right ventricle and a left bundle supplying the left ventricle.

Bundle branch block is present when either the right or the left bundle is unable to conduct. The depolarization wave then reaches the affected ventricular muscle by a different, slower pathway through the ventricular muscle.

CRITERIA FOR DIAGNOSIS OF BUNDLE BRANCH BLOCK

1   Prolonged QRS complex to 0·12 sec or more—because of slower spread of the depolarization wave through the myocardium distal to the block.

2   Abnormal shape of QRS complex—the depolarization wave takes an abnormal pathway, and the electrical forces generated by the heart are therefore abnormal in magnitude and direction.

RIGHT BUNDLE BRANCH BLOCK

Criteria (Fig. 1.22)

1   QRS 0·12 sec or more in duration.

2   S wave in lead 1.
3   RSR′ wave in V1.
All three criteria must be present to make the diagnosis.

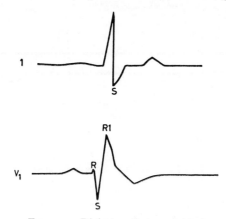

FIG. 1.22   Right bundle branch block

Mechanism

1   The prolonged QRS is a result of slower spread of the depolarization wave distal to the block.
2, 3   The right ventricle is depolarized last in right bundle branch block, because there is a delay in the depolarization impulse reaching the right ventricle. The right ventricle lies anterior to the left ventricle and the terminal forces of the QRS are therefore, directed anteriorly, producing an R′ in V1. The right ventricle also lies to the right of the left ventricle and the terminal forces of the QRS are therefore directed rightwards producing a terminal S wave in lead 1.

Causes

1   Normal variant. No cardiac abnormality is found in 15% of patients with right bundle branch block.
2   Right ventricular dilatation and hypertrophy, e.g. pulmonary embolism; atrial septal defect.
3   Ischaemic heart disease affecting the right bundle.
4   Following surgical ventriculotomy.

LEFT BUNDLE BRANCH BLOCK

Criteria (Fig. 1.23)

1   QRS 0·12 sec or more in duration.
2   Absent Q waves in V4, V5 and V6.
3   Absent R waves in V1.

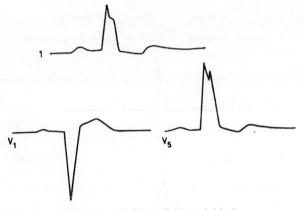

FIG. 1.23   Left bundle branch block

Mechanism
1   The prolonged QRS is a result of slow intramyocardial spread of depolarization beyond the block.
2, 3   Normally the interventricular septum is activated first and is depolarized from the left side, producing small Q waves in V4, V5 and V6 and a small R wave in V1. In left bundle branch block the interventricular septum is activated from the right bundle and depolarization spreads from the right side. This initial force is directed posteriorly and to the left and does not therefore write R waves in the anterior precordial leads V1 and V2, or Q waves in leads V4, V5 and V6.

Causes
Left bundle branch block implies heart disease e.g. myocardial ischaemia; cardiomyopathy; myocardial fibrosis.

Myocardial infarction
Myocardial infarction is in practice virtually confined to the left ventricle.

CRITERIA (Fig. 1.24)
1   ST segment elevation—within minutes of interference with coronary flow.
2   Q waves 0·04 sec or greater in width—appear within hours usually.
3   T wave inversion. The T waves become inverted in the leads showing ST elevation, and within a few weeks the ST segment becomes iso-electric.

The situation of the infarct determine the leads in which these changes are seen.

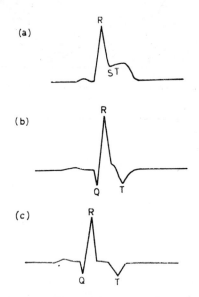

FIG. 1.24   Lead II   Inferior myocardial infarction:
(a)   2 hours after onset of pain
(b)   12 hours after onset of pain
(c)   2 weeks after onset

MECHANISM

ST segment elevation
A small current arises from injured cells in the ischaemic myocardium. This current of injury displaces the whole electrocardiogram downwards except during inscription of the ST segment, because the injury current does not flow during this brief period of complete depolarization. The effect is to give the impression of ST segment elevation.

0·04 sec Q waves
The arrows (Fig. 1.25, normal) represent the electrical forces during the initial .0·04 sec of ventricular depolarization (the ventricle is depolarized from the endocardial surface outwards). The large arrow is the average direction and magnitude of all these forces and normally does not vary much from the direction shown. Consider Fig. 1.25, inferior myocardial infarction.

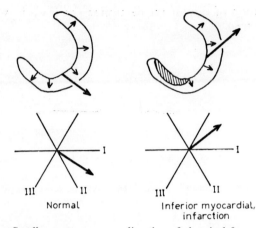

Normal   Inferior myocardial, infarction

FIG. 1.25   Small arrows represent direction of electrical forces in the left ventricle during the first 0·04 sec of ventricular depolarization. Larger arrow represents average direction of all forces during the first 0·04 sec

Myocardial infarction has involved the inferior aspect of the left ventricle and no electrical forces are produced in the necrotic area. The large arrow represents the average of the remaining initial 0·04 sec forces. This particular force will produce negative deflections in leads II and III during the first 0·04 sec of the QRS complex. Therefore inferior myocardial infarction produces Q waves lasting 0·04 sec in leads II and III. Similarly an anterior myocardial infarction will abolish all anteriorly directed forces during the initial 0·04 sec. Q waves in V1, V2 and V3 are the result, because there are now no initial anterior forces to produce R waves in these leads.

Fig. 1.26 shows the various locations of myocardial infarction.

Inversion of T waves

The direction of the repolarization wave in the ventricular muscle is altered, both by the presence of an area of muscle not taking part in this process (the infarcted area) and by abnormal repolarization of ischaemic muscle around the infarcted area.

T inversion is seen in the same leads that have Q waves.

SUMMARY OF THE ELECTROCARDIOGRAPHIC DIAGNOSIS OF INFARCTION

1   Pathological Q waves are produced by muscle necrosis. The presence of 0·04 sec Q waves is therefore reliable evidence of myocardial infarction.

2   ST segment elevation is produced by acute ischaemia but is also

caused by pericarditis. Serial electrocardiograms may show the development of Q waves and confirm infarction. Without these the diagnosis is uncertain.

3 T wave abnormalities. T wave changes alone are not diagnostic of infarction, abnormal T waves being found in many conditions—metabolic upsets, hypothyroidism, pericarditis, hypertrophy of the ventricle etc.

4 Bundle branch block and hemi-block (pp. 96, 280). Conduction abnormalities are common in myocardial infarction but not confined to this condition. The finding of bundle branch block or hemi-block is not diagnostic of myocardial infarction.

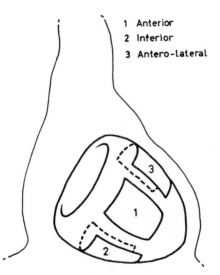

1 Anterior
2 Inferior
3 Antero-lateral

FIG. 1.26 Diagram of the left ventricle showing approximate locations of myocardial infarction

Abnormalities of the ST segment

Deviation of the ST segment more than 1 mm above or below the iso-electric line usually indicates disease.

CAUSES OF ST ELEVATION

1 Current of injury during the acute phase of infarction. Persistent ST elevation months after infarction is suggestive of ventricular aneurysm.

2 Acute pericarditis. ST segment elevation usually seen in many leads.

C

3   Healthy young adults with large upright T waves may have ST elevation in the leads with the tallest T waves.

CAUSES OF ST DEPRESSION

1   Digitalis effect. ST segment runs obliquely downwards, often described as an ST sag.
2   Sub-endocardial ischaemia. Straight ST depression is commonly present during an attack of angina pectoris.
3   LV hypertrophy. QRS complexes are tall and T waves inverted.
4   Metabolic abnormalities. Low serum potassium in particular.

P Wave Abnormalities

P MITRALE

Criteria
P wave is notched and 0·12 sec or more in duration (Fig. 1.27).

Mechanism
An enlarged left atrium produces P mitrale because depolarization of the left atrium takes longer when the size of the atrium is increased. The terminal part of the P wave represents left atrial depolarization and this terminal component is prolonged when the left atrium is large.

Causes
Mitral stenosis or incompetence.
Enlargement of the left atrium from other causes, e.g. hypertensive heart disease.

P PULMONALE

Criteria
P wave 2·5 mm or more in height and triangular in shape (Fig. 1.27).

Mechanism
The right atrium is hypertrophied and the electrical forces generated during right atrial depolarization are therefore increased. The P wave is not prolonged since the terminal component of the P wave, due to left atrial depolarisation, is not altered.

Causes
Right atrial hypertrophy, e.g. tricuspid stenosis; pulmonary stenosis; tricuspid atresia.

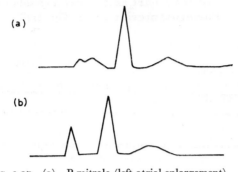

FIG. 1.27 (a) P mitrale (left atrial enlargement)
(b) P pulmonale (right atrial hypertrophy)

Abnormalities of Cardiac Rhythm

The electrocardiogram is of great value in the diagnosis of abnormal cardiac rhythms. The site of the impulse formation and the spread of this impulse through the myocardium can be ascertained. Lead II and precordial lead VI usually record P waves clearly and these leads are particularly useful in the diagnosis of arrhythmias (see pp. 88 *et seq*).

CHEST RADIOGRAPHY

The chest X-ray is used in heart disease for an assessment of the size of the individual chambers of the heart, the effects of the disease on the lungs, and the detection of calcium in the heart valves, pericardium and aorta.

Films Taken

Postero-anterior chest X-ray
Taken with a tube to patient distance of 6 feet, to minimize distortion.

Penetrated postero-anterior and penetrated left lateral chest X-rays
These penetrated films are valuable for the detection of calcium.

Oblique films with barium swallow, and other special views
Only used in special circumstances as usually all information available from the X-ray is obtainable from the postero-anterior and lateral films.

Contour of the Heart and Great Vessels on the Postero-Anterior Film (Fig. 1.28)

Right border

SUPERIOR VENA CAVA

Seen as a vertical line at the upper part of the right border between the sterno-clavicular region and the heart.

ASCENDING AORTA

A dilated ascending aorta projects to the right and distorts the normal smooth line of the superior vena cava e.g. post stenotic dilation due to aortic valve disease, aneurysm of the ascending aorta. Calcification of the ascending aorta suggests syphilitic aortitis.

RIGHT ATRIUM

The right atrium forms the lower part of the right border, from the termination of the superior vena cava to the diaphragm. A prominent or bulging right border of the heart may be due to right atrial enlargement (tricuspid valve disease, congestive heart failure) or Enlargement of the right ventricle displacing the normal right atrium or Pericardial effusion. These three causes cannot always be differentiated by their X-ray appearances alone.

Left border

AORTIC ARCH

The arch of the aorta is seen as a rounded knuckle at the upper left margin of the cardiac silhouette. The aortic knuckle is abnormally prominent in aortic incompetence or other lesions causing generalized dilatation of the aorta. Arteriosclerosis is a frequent cause of a prominent aortic knuckle, when a line of calcium in the aortic wall is often visible.

An inconspicuous aortic knuckle is characteristic of a chronic low cardiac output state e.g. severe mitral stenosis, large septal defects.

PULMONARY ARTERY

Immediately below the bulge of the aortic knuckle is a slight bulge on the left border of the heart produced by the normal pulmonary artery. An abnormally prominent pulmonary artery bulge indicates an enlarged main pulmonary artery due to:

1 Post stenotic dilatation of the pulmonary artery (pulmonary valve stenosis).

2 Increased flow through the pulmonary artery (atrial septal defect, ventricular septal defect, persistent ductus arteriosus).

3 Increased pressure in the pulmonary artery (pulmonary hypertension).

An inconspicuous pulmonary artery suggests either an abnormally small main pulmonary artery (Fallot's Tetralogy) or an absent pulmonary artery (pulmonary atresia).

LEFT ATRIAL APPENDAGE

Immediately below the pulmonary artery lies the left atrial appendage and enlargement of this produces a prominence on the cardiac border in this region. An atrial appendage of normal size is not visible on the chest X-ray.

Enlargement of the left atrium accompanies enlargement of its appendage and the enlarged atrium can be seen as a central shadow. The right border of this shadow is easily detected as a curved area of increased density within the shadow of the right atrium (8).

Radiological evidence of left atrial enlargement is provided by:

1 Enlargement of the atrial appendage.

2 Prominent right border of left atrium seen through the shadow of the right atrium.

3 Upward displacement of the left main bronchus.

4 Backward displacement of a barium filled oesophagus in the right anterior oblique view—rarely necessary as the other signs are usually obvious.

VENTRICLE

Normally the left ventricle forms the left lower part of the cardiac silhouette and dilatation of this chamber displaces the lower left border of the heart to the left. Dilatation of the right ventricle, however, also displaces the lower left cardiac border outwards and the chest X-ray is not reliable in the differentiation of right from left ventricular enlargement.

An enlarged heart is judged to be present when the widest transverse diameter of the heart is more than half the widest internal diameter of the thorax (cardio-thoracic ratio greater than 0·5). The determination of which chamber is causing the enlargement is best achieved from the electrocardiogram. Ventricular hypertrophy without dilatation cannot be assessed from the X-ray.

The Lung Fields

Cardiovascular disease may alter the appearance of the lung fields in five main ways:

Increased pulmonary blood flow (pulmonary plethora)

The vascular lung markings are larger, more numerous and extend far out to the periphery. The larger branches of the pulmonary arteries and the main pulmonary veins are responsible for normal lung markings and these vessels dilate and smaller branches become visible when flow through the lungs is increased. Pulmonary plethora indicates a left to right cardiac shunt.

Increased pulmonary vascular resistance (pulmonary hypertension)

The proximal pulmonary arteries are large but the peripheral vessels become almost invisible leaving the peripheral lung fields abnormally clear and translucent. The high pulmonary arterial pressure accounts for the dilatation of the main pulmonary artery and the proximal branches, and the intense constriction of the smaller pulmonary arteries renders the vascular markings less obvious at the periphery.

Decreased pulmonary blood flow (oligaemic lung fields)

The vascular markings are small and sparse and the lung fields are abnormally clear. Oligaemic lung fields are seen in: pulmonary stenosis; Fallot's tetralogy; tricuspid atresia; pulmonary atresia.

Pulmonary venous congestion (caused by pulmonary venous hypertension)

The pulmonary veins are dilated and more easily seen, and there is increased tissue fluid in the interstitial tissues of the lung which produces:

1 An overall ground glass appearance of the lung fields.
2 A peri-hilar flare from increased lung density around the hilum.
3 Fine horizontal straight lines 3–5 mm in length, best seen in the lower lung fields in the costo-phrenic angles (Kerley B lines). These are the result of oedema of the interlobular septa of the lungs.

Pulmonary oedema

This represents extreme pulmonary venous hypertension (over 40 mm Hg.). At this level the alveoli fill with fluid and patchy shadowing of the lungs due to areas of oedema-filled lung are seen, particularly around the hila and extending out into the surrounding lung.

Detection of Calcium in the Heart

Screening of the heart using an image intensifier is a very satisfactory way of detecting calcium in the heart, but properly penetrated postero-anterior and left lateral X-rays of the heart subject the patient to a much smaller dosage of radiation and are almost as informative.

Calcification in the heart valves

Mitral valve calcification when present is seen on the penetrated postero-anterior chest X-ray rather lower than calcium in the aortic valve. In Fig. 1.28, 10 represents the area where calcium of the mitral valve is seen. In the lateral view mitral valve calcification is seen in the posterior third of the cardiac shadow.

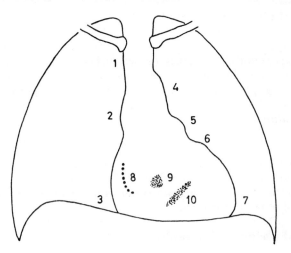

FIG. 1.28   Skiagram of the chest: cardiac contours:

1	Superior vena cava	7	Left ventricle
2	Ascending aorta	8	Margin of left atrium lying behind the right atrium
3	Right atrial border		
4	Aortic knuckle	9	Position of aortic valve calcium
5	Main pulmonary artery	10	Position of mitral valve calcium
6	Left atrial appendage—only visible when enlarged		

Aortic valve calcification is seen on the postero-anterior film in the region marked 9 in Fig. 1.28 and in the lateral view in the middle third of the heart shadow.

Calcification of the pericardium

Calcification of the pericardium may be obvious as a dense ring surrounding the heart in the postero-anterior chest X-ray but, when less marked, it may best be demonstrated on a penetrated lateral view.

SPECIAL METHODS OF INVESTIGATION USED IN SELECTED CASES

Phonocardiography

A phonocardiogram is a graphic recording of the heart sounds and murmurs. The recording site may either be the chest wall (external phonocardiography) or from within the heart (internal phonocardiography).

External phonocardiography

TECHNIQUE
The heart sounds and murmurs are picked up by a microphone attached to the chest wall and recorded as a series of vibrations on fast moving photographic film. The electrocardiogram and the carotid arterial pulsation are recorded simultaneously to aid in the identification of the sounds.

USES
As a means of checking the information obtained on auscultation, particularly for the accurate timing of heart sounds and murmurs. The external phonocardiogram is not as sensitive as the ear in the detection of faint murmurs.

Internal phonocardiography

TECHNIQUE
A very small microphone is inserted into the cardiac chambers on the tip of a cardiac catheter and the sounds recorded on a photographic film.

USES
Some murmurs can be localized to the individual chambers in which they occur, and externally inaudible murmurs can be recorded.

Apex Cardiography

The apex cardiogram is a recording of the movement of the skin overlying the apex beat throughout the cardiac cycle. It amplifies the information obtained by clinical palpation.

Technique

The instrument consists of a wide ring containing a small metal probe in its centre. The ring is held against the chest wall so that the movements of the cardiac apex beat displace the probe upwards and downwards and this movement is amplified and recorded electrically on fast-moving photographic film (Fig. 1.29).

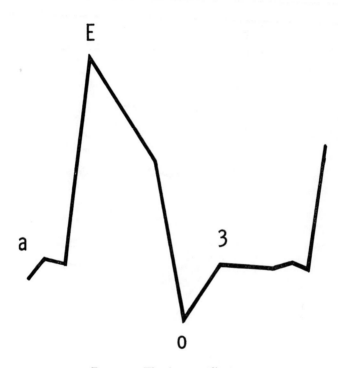

FIG. 1.29   The Apex cardiogram

Value of apex cardiogram

1   Identifies sounds when recorded simultaneously with the phonocardiogram. o point corresponds closely to opening of mitral valve and to the opening snap. 3 ends the rapid filling phase and coincides with a 3rd heart sound.

2   Reveals early signs of left ventricular stress. The *a* wave is caused by left atrial systole and is less than 10% of the total deflection in normals. An *a* wave greater than 10% may be present in ischaemic heart disease, hypertensive heart disease and cardiomyopathy.

Ultrasound (Echocardiography) (Fig. 1.30)

The instrument held against the chest wall projects a beam of sound through the heart. Echoes are obtained from the anterior leaf of the mitral valve, as in the drawing, but echoes are also reflected from the right ventricle, interventricular septum, left ventricle and pericardium.

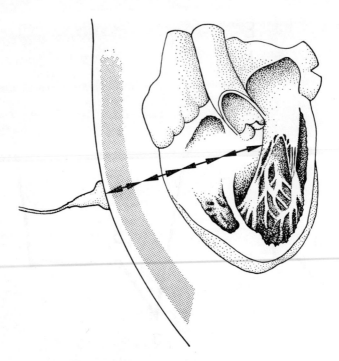

FIG. 1.30   Ultrasound (Echocardiography)

Value of Ultrasound

1   Mitral stenosis.

The diastolic closure rate of the anterior leaf of the mitral valve as measured by ultrasound is always well below 70 mm per second in significant mitral stenosis. Multiple strong echoes indicate mitral valve calcification.

2   Pericardial effusion.

The presence and size of an effusion is determined accurately.

3   Left atrial myxoma.

Characteristic echo obtained from the tumour.

4 Diagnostic or strongly suggestive echoes obtained in hypertrophic obstructive cardiomyopathy, tricuspid valve abnormalities, mitral atresia and acute severe aortic regurgitation.

Cardiac Catheterization and Angiocardiography

Objects
1 Pressure measurements are made within the cardiac chambers and great vessels.
2 Samples of blood are obtained from the cardiac chambers and great vessels and are analysed for their oxygen content and their percentage oxygen saturation.
3 Radio-opaque contrast fluid can be injected directly into any cardiac chamber, and the subsequent passage of this fluid through the heart outlines the anatomy of the chambers and great vessels on serially exposed X-ray films, or on cine film.

Techniques

RIGHT HEART CATHETERIZATION
The cardiac catheter is passed through a vein in the arm or leg into the right atrium, then onwards under X-ray control through the right ventricle and pulmonary artery until the tip wedges in a small pulmonary artery. The pressure in this wedged position closely corresponds to the pressure in the pulmonary veins. Samples and pressures can be taken from the pulmonary artery, right ventricle and right atrium as the catheter is withdrawn.

LEFT HEART CATHETERIZATION

Retrograde approach
The catheter is placed in the femoral or brachial artery and advanced to the aortic valve and through it to the left ventricle.

Trans-septal approach
The catheter is advanced from the femoral vein to the right atrium, then through the atrial septum into the left atrium and through the mitral valve to the left ventricle. Either a patent foramen ovale is used or the atrial septum is punctured by a needle passed up the inside of the catheter.

The choice between these two methods largely depends on the lesion being investigated e.g. the trans-septal method is the best approach to the left ventricle when there is stenosis of the aortic valve.

ANGIOCARDIOGRAPHY

Radio-opaque contrast solution, such as 85% hypaque is injected under pressures of over 100 lb/in² through a catheter into the heart. Usually about 1 ml/Kg body weight is injected into whichever cardiac chamber is to be studied in detail.

High-speed cine cameras record the passage of the injected contrast fluid at over 60 frames per sec, or up to 12 full-size films per sec can be obtained in two planes simultaneously with special radiographic equipment.

General indications and value

CONFIRMATION OF THE CLINICAL DIAGNOSIS

Septal defects
There is a rise in oxygen saturation of samples taken from the chamber into which the left to right shunt occurs, and this rise is maintained in all chambers beyond. The catheter can often be passed across the defect.

Valve stenosis
A high pressure is found in the chamber on the proximal side of a narrowed valve and a low pressure immediately beyond the obstruction. Angiocardiography demonstrates the anatomy of the obstruction.

Valve incompetence
At angiocardiography radio-opaque contrast is injected into the chamber beyond the leaking valve and is seen to regurgitate across the damaged valve into a proximal chamber.

ESTIMATION OF THE SEVERITY OF THE LESION

Septal defects with left to right shunts
The size of the defect is estimated by the magnitude of the increase in oxygen content of the blood at the chamber involved in the shunt —a large increase implies a large shunt and, by inference, a large defect.

The pulmonary blood flow is obtained by measuring the oxygen uptake by the lungs per minute and dividing this by the difference in oxygen content between the samples taken from a pulmonary vein and the pulmonary artery:

$$\text{Pulmonary blood flow} = \frac{\text{Oxygen uptake}}{\text{Pulmonary venous} - \text{Pulmonary arterial}}$$
$$\text{oxygen content} \quad \text{oxygen content}$$

The effect of the shunt on the pulmonary arterioles is measured by the pulmonary vascular resistance:

$$\text{Pulmonary vascular resistance} = \frac{\text{Mean pulmonary} - \text{Mean pulmonary}}{\text{Pulmonary blood flow}}$$
$$\text{artery pressure} \quad \text{venous pressure}$$

Valve stenosis
A narrowed valve offers resistance to blood flow and the pressure is therefore higher in the chamber proximal to the stenosis. The size of the stenotic valve orifice is calculated from a knowledge of the pressure drop across the valve and the rate of blood flow across the valve. Thus:

$$\text{Aortic orifice area (cm}^2) = \frac{\text{Mean systolic flow}}{44 \cdot 5 \sqrt{\text{mean pressure gradient}}}$$

Valve incompetence
The severity of the regurgitation can be graded mild, moderate or severe from the angiocardiogram, according to the observed degree of reflux of contrast medium across the damaged valve.

DEMONSTRATION OF THE ANATOMY OF THE LESION
When this is necessary, it is best done by angiocardiography.

DEMONSTRATION OR EXCLUSION OF ADDITIONAL LESIONS
Any severe cardiac lesion may obscure the clinical signs of additional lesions e.g. in the presence of a large ventricular septal defect with pulmonary hypertension, a persistent ductus arteriosus cannot be excluded by clinical examination.

Atrial septal defect is commonly complicated by anomalous pulmonary veins draining into the right atrium, often not appreciable on the chest X-ray.

Cardiac catheterization and angiocardiography will reveal these additional lesions.

Complications of cardiac catheterization and angiocardiography

The mortality from right heart catheterization is less than $0 \cdot 1\%$

unless very ill infants are being investigated in whom the risk is substantially greater. Angiocardiography carries a slightly increased risk and left heart catheterization with angiocardiography has the highest complication rate—mortality approaches 0·5%. The list of possible complications includes:

1   Production of atrial and ventricular arrhythmias, including ventricular fibrillation.
2   Pulmonary embolism during right heart catheterization.
3   Systemic embolism during left heart catheterization.
4   Puncture of the heart by catheter, causing tamponade.
5   Injection of radio-opaque fluid into the myocardium.

CHAPTER 2
COMPLICATIONS OF HEART DISEASE

(a) HEART FAILURE

Definition

Heart failure is a condition in which ventricular output is able to match the venous return only after a substantial increase in filling pressure has occurred.

Types
Left ventricular failure.
Right ventricular failure.
Congestive cardiac failure (combined right and left ventricular failure).

Causes

PRESSURE OVERLOAD
The work of the ventricle is increased when it is required to work against an increased pressure.

VOLUME OVERLOAD
The work of the ventricle is increased when it is required to give an abnormally high volume output.

VENTRICULAR MUSCLE DISEASE
The myocardium may be abnormal secondarily to coronary artery disease, or as a result of primary disease of the heart muscle (cardio-myopathy).

Disturbance of Physiology in Cardiac Failure

The diastolic pressure and volume of the failing ventricle is increased. The cardiac output is usually low and fails to increase normally during exertion. Sodium and water are retained by the kidneys with consequent increase in total body extra-cellular fluid.

Mechanism

RAISED DIASTOLIC PRESSURE AND VOLUME

The force of ventricular contraction can be increased principally in two ways—Increase in length of ventricular muscle fibres at the end of diastole; Increased activity of the sympathetic nervous system.

When the length and tension of the fibres of a failing ventricle are increased in diastole a more powerful systolic contraction can be obtained, i.e. the ventricle works from a greater end-diastolic pressure and volume.

The sympathetic nervous system is also used to augment the force of ventricular contraction and the level of circulating catecholamines is increased in heart failure.

LOW CARDIAC OUTPUT

Despite these compensatory mechanisms the ventricle expels only a fraction of its contents at each beat and the cardiac output is low.

SODIUM AND WATER RETENTION

Factors involved

Reduced renal blood flow and glomeruler filtration rate as a consequence of a low cardiac output.

Excessive reabsorption of sodium by the renal tubules, possibly influenced by some hormone with properties similar to aldosterone. Aldosterone itself is not always present in excess in heart failure nor is any mechanism known whereby heart failure could produce an excess of aldosterone.

Left Ventricular Failure

Causes

1   Pressure overload (aortic stenosis, systemic hypertension).

2   Volume overload (aortic incompetence, mitral incompetence, persistent ductus arteriosus).

3   Myocardial disease (myocardial infarction, cardiomyopathy, endomyocardial fibrosis).

Symptoms

Produced by the high pulmonary venous pressure and the excess of sodium and water in the lungs:

1   Increased dyspnoea on exertion.

2   Orthopnoea.

3 Paroxysmal nocturnal dyspnoea.
4 Acute dyspnoea accompanied by frothy sputum (pulmonary oedema).
5 Cough, haemoptysis, respiratory tract infections.

Clinical signs

GENERAL
Patient seated upright in bed unable to lie flat and respiratory rate increased. Cyanosis is absent until pulmonary oedema develops.

ARTERIAL PULSE
Sinus tachycardia (probably due to increased sympathetic activity).
    Pulsus alternans—Alternate strong and weak left ventricular contractions best detected by the sphygmomanometer.

JUGULAR VENOUS PRESSURE
Slight elevation above the sternal angle (increased blood volume produced by sodium and water retention).

CARDIAC IMPULSES
Apex beat displaced outside the mid clavicular line (dilatation of the failing ventricle).
    Palpable third heart sound.

AUSCULTATION
Third heart sound at the apex indicating left ventricular failure (p. 29).

LUNGS
Fine crepitations at lung bases (fluid in bronchioles as a result of high pressure in the pulmonary veins).
    Widespread crepitations, coarse râles and rhonchi may be heard during an attack of pulmonary oedema (fluid in alveoli and bronchi with super-imposed bronchial spasm).
    The absence of basal crepitations does not completely exclude the diagnosis of left ventricular failure—considerable congestion of the lungs may be present in some patients without excessive fluid in the bronchi.

Electrocardiogram
The electrocardiogram gives no information on the force of contraction of the heart and can be normal in severe failure. Usually the electrocardiogram shows changes of the underlying lesion which has

been responsible for the failure, e.g. left ventricular hypertrophy
suggests an increased pressure or volume load; evidence of myocardial infarction will point to coronary artery disease; broad
abnormal QRS complexes and abnormalities of rhythm favour the
diagnosis of cardiomyopathy, but are also frequent in ischaemic
heart disease.

Chest X-ray
Increased transverse diameter of the heart (dilated left ventricle).
Evidence of pulmonary venous congestion (p. 56).

Right Ventricular Failure

Causes
1 Pressure overload—pulmonary stenosis, pulmonary hypertension.
2 Volume overload—atrial septal defect, tricuspid incompetence.
3 Myocardial disease—endomyocardial fibrosis, amyloid disease.

Symptoms
Produced by a low cardiac output, elevated systemic venous pressure
and accumulation of oedema fluid in the tissues. Breathlessness is not
prominent and orthopnoea and paroxysmal dyspnoea do not occur
(pulmonary venous congestion absent):
1 Fatigue (low cardiac output).
2 Epigastric pain and abdominal fullness (enlarged, congested
liver).
3 Swelling of ankles (the oedema of cardiac failure drains to the
lower limbs under the influence of gravity).

Clinical signs

JUGULAR VENOUS PULSE
Considerably elevated above the sternal angle (filling pressure of the
right ventricle increased).

CARDIAC IMPULSES
1 Heave to left of sternum (enlarged right ventricle).
2 Apex beat may be outside the mid-clavicular line and formed by
the greatly enlarged right ventricle.
3 Palpable third sound.

AUSCULTATION
1 Pansystolic murmur to left of lower sternum (functional tricuspid
incompetence, a result of dilatation of the tricuspid valve).

2   Third heart sound in same region, indicating right ventricular failure.

LUNGS
Signs of small pleural effusion.

LIVER
Enlarged, tender (distended by increased systemic venous pressure transmitted via the hepatic veins).

OEDEMA
Excess body sodium and water collecting in the tissues and serous cavaties:
1   Pitting oedema of ankles.
2   Pad of sacral oedema in patients confined to bed.
3   Pleural effusion, ascites.

Electrocardiogram
Right ventricular hypertrophy usually present because prolonged strain on the right ventricle is the usual cause of right ventricular failure.

Chest X-ray
1   Increased transverse diameter of the heart (dilated right ventricle).
2   Lung fields normal unless pulmonary infarction occurs (the sluggish circulation of right ventricular failure favours thrombus formation in the leg veins).
3   Pleural effusion (if present usually small).

Congestive Cardiac Failure

Right ventricular failure is commonly secondary to left ventricular failure, the high venous pressure in the pulmonary veins increasing the pulmonary artery pressure and overburdening the right ventricle. This combination of right and left ventricular failure, with symptoms and signs of both, is called congestive cardiac failure.

Heart Failure in Infancy

The criteria for the diagnosis of heart failure in infancy are different, the history being that of feeding difficulties rather than dyspnoea, and the liver size is used as an estimate of the venous congestion since the jugular venous pressure is not readily visible.

Criteria

1 History of feeding difficulties—frequent pauses during the feed, lack of strength to take the feed.
2 Tachypnoea—evidence of difficulty in breathing.
3 Tachycardia.
4 Hepatomegaly.
5 Oedema—often generalized, including the face.
6 Chest X-ray evidence of an enlarged heart.
7 Failure to gain weight—chronic cases.

(b) BACTERIAL ENDOCARDITIS

Definition

Bacterial invasion of a heart valve or of an area of endocardium. There are two types, depending on the virulence of the invading organism—acute bacterial endocarditis; subacute bacterial endocarditis.

Acute Bacterial Endocarditis

During an acute septicaemia with virulent organisms such as *Staph. aureus*, *gonococcus*, or *Strep. pyogenes*, previously normal heart valves may be invaded and rapidly destroyed. The clinical picture is that of an acute septicaemia and the course of the illness a few weeks.

Subacute Bacterial Endocarditis

Aetiology

Organisms of low grade virulence only invade a valve or an area of endocardium that has been damaged by previous acquired disease, such as rheumatic fever, or is the site of turbulent blood flow due to a congenital cardiac defect. The endocardium in the proximity of a turbulent flow is readily invaded by organisms because its nutrition from the blood stream is poor. Congenital defects producing a high pressure jet of blood (small ventricular septal defects) are particularly prone to infection, whereas lesions causing little turbulence (atrial septal defects) are not so prone.

1 Common invading organisms:
Streptococcus viridans—60%
Streptococcus faecalis—10%
2 Lesions particularly liable to infection—mitral incompetence (especially mild mitral incompetence), aortic incompetence, small

ventricular septal defects, persistent ductus arteriosus, congenital bicuspid aortic valve, pulmonary valve stenosis, coarctation of aorta.

Mode of infection

Blood is normally sterile and any bacteria entering the blood stream are quickly killed by the normal body defences. Damaged endothelium allows them to survive and proliferate.

Bacteria enter the blood stream in the following circumstances, all of which can cause bacterial endocarditis:

1 *Streptococcus viridans* bacteraemia—dental extraction, extensive dental treatment, apical tooth abscess or even from chewing food with apparently normal teeth.

2 *Strep. faecalis*—instrumentation of the genito-urinary tract, diarrhoea.

3 Other bacteria—puerperal sepsis, osteomyelitis, operations on the large bowel.

Morbid anatomy

Bacteria invade the damaged valve or endocardium, and platelets, fibrin and bacteria form large friable vegetations in which the bacteria are protected both from the normal defence mechanisms and to some extent from antibiotics in the blood stream.

Complications

1 Valve incompetence results from destruction of endocardium and rupture of chordae tendineae. Discrete holes in valve tissue are particularly characteristic of bacterial endocarditis.

2 Embolic incidents occur when a fragment of the vegetations (usually a small fragment) becomes detached. Systemic embolism indicates vegetations on the left side of the heart, while pulmonary infarcts are found when pulmonary valve, ventricular septal defect or persistent ductus arteriosus is infected, because the emboli are carried to the lungs. The infarcts of subacute bacterial endocarditis do not suppurate.

3 Mycotic aneurysms. Infection of the muscular wall of a medium sized artery following embolism may cause localized weakening and aneurysm formation. Occasionally these aneurysms rupture.

Clinical presentation

In the presence of a cardiac lesion capable of becoming infected any unexplained fever or period of ill health suggests the possibility of subacute bacterial endocarditis. Recent dental treatment precedes an attack in 50% of cases.

SYMPTOMS (DUE TO TOXAEMIA, EMBOLISM AND
HEART FAILURE)

1 Toxaemic symptoms—malaise, anorexia, weight loss, excessive
perspiration and shivering at night.
2 Embolic symptoms:
     (i) Attacks of abdominal pain (splenic, renal or mesenteric in-
farct).
     (ii) Hemiplegia, monoplegia, loss of vision in one eye (cerebral
embolism).
     (iii) Chest pain, haemoptysis (pulmonary infarcts).
3 Heart failure. Dyspnoea, orthopnoea and oedema appear when
cardiac failure follows increased valve damage.

CLINICAL EXAMINATION

1 Signs due to an infective process.
     (i) Pyrexia, usually low grade and intermittent.
     (ii) Pale complexion with underlying brown discolouration due
mainly to the early development of anaemia.
     (iii) Multiple capillary haemorrhages under the nails (splinter
haemorrhages).
     (iv) Finger clubbing within six weeks of onset of symptoms in over
half the cases.
     (v) Splenomegaly (small and soft in early cases, large and firm in
chronic cases).
2 Embolic signs.
     (i) Osler's nodes (cutaneous emboli). Small, tender, erythematous
swellings found on the pads of the fingers and toes, sides of the fingers
and on the thenar and hypothenar eminences.
     (ii) Deeper swellings (infected emboli). Red tender swellings up
to the size of an orange, anywhere on the limb. Suppuration does not
occur.
     (iii) Retinal emboli—haemorrhages with white centres in the
optic fundus.
     (iv) Red cells in the urine—focal embolic glomerulo-nephritis
from multiple small bacterial emboli into the glomerular capillaries,
some of which are destroyed with consequent escape of red cells into
the urine.
     (v) Absent pulsation in a smaller artery such as the posterior tibial
or radial artery (embolism of that vessel).
3 Signs in the heart. The murmurs of a lesion predisposing to
bacterial endocarditis are usually present and can vary from day to
day as destruction of tissue continues. If the underlying lesion is a
congenital bicuspid aortic valve the heart may be normal on clinical
examination.

INVESTIGATIONS

1 Blood culture. Isolation of the infecting organism is vital to proper treatment and a positive blood culture can be obtained from at least 80% of cases. Antibiotics are therefore not given until at least three blood cultures have been set up. It is unlikely that a positive culture will be obtained if three initial cultures are negative. In the absence of a positive blood culture there is always some doubt about the diagnosis and about the choice of antibiotic for therapy.

2 Blood. The peripheral blood shows an elevated erythrocyte sedimentation rate, progressive normocytic normochromic anaemia, and a mild leucocytosis.

3 Urine. The urine contains red cells on microscopy.

Prognosis
Bacteriological cure can be obtained in nearly every case. Unfortunately the five-year cure rate is usually less than 50%, with patients dying from renal complications or severe valve damage.

Prophylaxis
In all patients having cardiac lesions liable to infection, antibiotics are given to cover the following procedures:

Dental extraction or dental scaling, tonsillectomy, bronchoscopy, instrumentation of the genito-urinary tract, childbirth, surgery of the lower intestinal tract.

Recommended antibiotic cover for dental therapy is 600,000 units crystalline penicillin combined with 600,000 units procaine penicillin given intramuscularly 1 hour before the operation, continuing with procaine penicillin 600,000 units daily for two days. For patients sensitive to penicillin, cephaloridine 500 mg intra-muscularly immediately prior to dental extraction followed by oral erythromycin estolate 250 mg q.d.s. is recommended. For instrumentation of the genito-urinary tract crystalline penicillin 1 mega unit is given intra-muscularly 30 minutes before the operation, together with ampicillin 250 mg q.d.s. for 2 days by mouth.

Treatment of subacute bacterial endocarditis
The disease is invariably fatal unless the infecting organism is completely eradicated by the administration of an appropriate antibiotic.

CHOICE OF ANTIBIOTIC

Bactericidal antibiotics must be used in high dosage and for long periods (at least 6 weeks). The best antibiotic to use is determined from the results of sensitivity tests on the organism cultured from the blood. The bacteriological laboratory can given an initial report within 24 hours on the antibiotics which inhibit growth of the organism, and over the course of the next few days further *in vitro* tests are performed to confirm that the suggested antibiotic is bactericidal at concentrations that can be achieved in the patient's blood.

Penicillin is usually the drug of choice for *Strep. viridans* infections, and very large doses of penicillin with some other bactericidal antibiotic such as streptomycin or ampicillin are used for *Strep. faecalis* infections or when blood cultures have been negative. There is little hope of curing the patient unless a bactericidal antibiotic can be used.

DOSAGE

The blood level should be maintained at approximately four times the *in vitro* bactericidal level for the cultured organism. When penicillin is used the intramuscular route is preferred for dosages up to 20 mega units a day. Higher dosages than this are best given intravenously. Oral therapy should not be used as absorption of penicillin from the gastro-intestinal tract is unreliable and variable.

SURGERY

The appearance of severe heart failure strongly suggests acute aortic or acute mitral regurgitation. Acute aortic regurgitation is badly tolerated and, if heart failure does not respond to medical therapy within a few days, aortic valve replacement in the acute stage of the illness is life saving.

Diagnosis may be difficult because the characteristic early diastolic murmur is not heard. The pulse is small and sharp, there is a loud gallop rhythm with a soft first heart sound. Ultrasound shows closure of the mitral valve early in diastole.

DENTAL TREATMENT

Antibiotic therapy quickly leads to resistant organisms replacing the normal flora of the mouth and any dental treatment should be done immediately or as early as practicable in the treatment period. Steroids and anticoagulants play no part in the treatment of bacterial endocarditis.

EVALUATION OF THERAPY

On about the fourth day of treatment the patient's serum, taken immediately before the next dose of antibiotic, is tested for its ability to kill the infecting organism. The therapy is adequate if a fourfold dilution of this serum proves bactericidal to the cultured organism.

(c) SYSTEMIC EMBOLISM

Aetiology

From heart or pulmonary veins.

Clot
From left ventricle (myocardial infarction) or left atrium (mitral stenosis and atrial fibrillation). 10–30% of patients with mitral stenosis have systemic embolism, the incidence varying with the size of the left atrial appendage (14% if small, 48% if large) and rhythm (three quarters of emboli are associated with atrial fibrillation). Mitral stenosis need not be severe (12% of emboli occur with trivial stenosis).

Infected thrombus
Subacute bacterial endocarditis of aortic and mitral valve.

Tumour tissue
Fragments of left atrial myxoma may impact in peripheral arteries.

Calcium, air, fibrin etc.
Particularly after cardiac operations on the left heart.

Paradoxical embolism
Venous emboli may reach the systemic circulation through a right to left shunt (e.g. Fallot's Tetralogy).

Clinical Presentation

The initiating lesion is usually apparent, except when it is a painless myocardial infarct.

Cerebral embolism (60%)
Abrupt onset of neurological deficit, often with rapid recovery.

Visceral embolism (10%)
1 Spleen—left hypochondriac pain and friction rub.
2 Kidneys—loin pain and haematuria.
3 Mesenteric arteries—acute abdomen, ileus and melaena.

Peripheral embolism (30%)

Sudden pain and loss of function of limb. Pallor, coldness, anaesthesia and absent pulses. Differentiated from thrombosis and atheromatous narrowing by the absence of a previous history of claudication etc.

Treatment

Cerebral embolism

1 Maintenance of cerebral blood flow by sustaining the blood pressure and treating heart failure (oxygen, digitalis etc.).
2 Anticoagulation for prevention of further emboli may do more harm from intracerebral bleeding than good from prevention of propagated thrombus in the brain, and should be delayed for 2–3 weeks.
3 Reduction of surrounding oedema with steroids (e.g. dexamethazone).

Visceral embolism

1 Splenic and renal embolism—conservative (as cerebral).
2 Mesenteric embolism—resection of gangrenous bowel or mesenteric embolectomy.

Peripheral embolism

CONSERVATIVE

If limb is clearly viable anticoagulation is begun with heparin, and continued with warfarin. Heart failure is treated if present. The limb is kept level (to prevent oedema), at room temperature (to lower oxygen demands), and the rest of the body is warmed with heat and whiskey (to cause reflex vasodilation of the limb).

EMBOLECTOMY

Indications

Almost always required for a saddle (aortic bifurcation) embolus, almost never for brachial embolus. In lower limb embolism, if the limb does not appear viable (still pale, cold, paralysed and anaesthetic) 6 hours after the onset, embolectomy is indicated.

Technique

An incision is made at or below the point where the pulse disappears. Proximal and distal clot is removed with a Fogarty (balloon tipped) catheter until bleeding is free from both ends, when the artery is sutured.

MITRAL VALVOTOMY AND LEFT ATRIAL APPENDECTOMY
If significant mitral stenosis is present, or if the left atrial appendage is large, an emergency mitral valvotomy and left atrial appendectomy is performed immediately before embolectomy. Recurrent embolism (60%) is thereby reduced.

(d) PULMONARY EMBOLISM

Definition

Pulmonary embolism results when the pulmonary artery or one of its branches becomes obstructed by a thrombus or other substance (fat, air, or foreign body) carried there by the blood stream.

Pulmonary Embolism due to Thrombus

Aetiology

ORIGIN
1   Deep veins of legs.
2   Ilio-femoral segment (superficial and common femoral and iliac veins). Usual source of large emboli.
3   Right heart (10% of pulmonary emboli).

Local injury to the vein
Inflammation or trauma, e.g. thrombophlebitis, leg fractures.

Slowing of blood flow through the veins
    General   Heart failure.
    Local   Venous obstruction by pregnancy, obesity, anomalous iliac arteries or pressure on calves in bed or on the operating table.

Increased tendency of blood to form thrombi
Particularly common after childbirth, surgical operations and widespread malignant disease, but also may complicate poly-cythaemia and dehydration.

Pathology
When part of the thrombus separates from the vein it is carried into the lungs where it impacts in a pulmonary artery. Subsequent changes depend on the size of the embolus.

MASSIVE PULMONARY EMBOLISM

Circulatory changes appear when 60–85% of the pulmonary arterial tree is occluded. The right ventricle dilates and contracts feebly. Cardiac output and venous return are abruptly reduced, explaining why the jugular venous and right ventricular pressures may be only slightly raised after the initial episode. Pulmonary infarction does not necessarily occur because some blood circumvents the obstruction and maintains the viability of the lung tissue with the help of the bronchial arteries.

PULMONARY INFARCTION

Smaller emboli cause no general circulatory disturbance but may result in necrosis of a wedge of pulmonary tissue, particularly if there is impairment of pulmonary circulation (chronic pulmonary venous congestion or after operation). The necrotic lung becomes stuffed with blood from the still patent bronchial circulation, and the overlying pleura becomes inflamed.

MULTIPLE PERIPHERAL EMBOLI

Showers of multiple small emboli may impact in the smaller peripheral pulmonary arteries. Particularly common in women after pregnancy, when widespread obstruction raises the resistance in the pulmonary arterial tree and produces chronic pulmonary hypertension and right ventricular strain (p. 308).

SILENT PULMONARY EMBOLISM

Pulmonary embolism of moderate sized thrombi frequently gives few indications that it has occurred.

Clinical presentation

DIAGNOSIS OF DEEP VEIN THROMBOSIS

Tenderness, swelling, increased temperature of one leg suggests deep vein thrombosis but clinical signs are usually absent.

Radioactive fibrinogen uptake following intravenous injection

This test reveals many cases by showing an unequal uptake in the lower limbs. Over 30% of patients with myocardial infarction are positive to this test.

Doppler Test

This detects obstruction in the proximal veins of the legs. A normal acceleration of blood flow is absent on massaging the affected leg.

MASSIVE EMBOLISM

Symptoms
Classically after using a bedpan (straining raises the venous pressure, dilates the veins and tends to dislodge thrombus), the patient collapses with dyspnoea (acutely lowered cardiac output affecting the respiratory centre via the carotid sinus) and chest pain (probably due to the overloaded right ventricle receiving a poor coronary supply as a result of the low cardiac output).

Clinical examination
   General   Collapse, unconsciousness, respiratory distress and peripheral cyanosis (acutely lowered cardiac output).
   Pulse and blood pressure   Tachycardia and hypotension (low cardiac output).
   Jugular venous pressure   Initially high but fails as the right ventricle fails and cardiac output and venous return fall.
   Cardiac impulses   Usually normal. Right ventricular hypertrophy suggests long standing rather than acute strain.
   Auscultation   Atrial (4th) sound (right atrial strain) and a 3rd sound, loudest on inspiration, at the left sternal edge (right ventricular failure). The pulmonary second sound is accentuated (raised pulmonary arterial pressure) and delayed (prolonged right ventricular ejection time).

Electrocardiography
Right axis deviation, or right bundle branch block and T wave inversion in leads V_{1-4} (acute right ventricular strain) may be seen but the electrocardiogram is usually normal.

Chest X-ray
Enlargement of proximal pulmonary arteries and ischaemia of peripheral vessels.

Cardiac catheterization
The right atrial, ventricular and pulmonary arterial pressures are raised though often only slightly (cardiac output and venous return are reduced).

Angiography
Injection of contrast medium into the pulmonary artery provides an accurate diagnosis and shows the site of the embolus.

Radio-isotope pulmonary scanning
Injection of radioactive tagged macro-albumen aggregates followed
by pulmonary scanning will show which areas of the lung are
ischaemic.

PULMONARY INFARCTION

Symptoms
Pleuritic pain (inflamed pleura over infarct) and haemoptysis of
bright red blood (bronchial arterial blood from infarct).

Clinical examination
Often negative, but tachypnoea and a pleural rub (inflamed pleura)
may occur, sometimes accompanied by a bloodstained pleural
effusion.

Chest X-ray
May be negative, but patchy opacities of any shape provide useful
confirmatory evidence (the classical wedge shape is rare). There may
be a pleural effusion. The pulmonary artery to the infarcted segment
is dilated, and the diaphragm on the affected side may be raised
(reflex decrease in ventilation of the underperfused segment).

MULTIPLE PERIPHERAL EMBOLISM

Presents as pulmonary hypertension (p. 83) with dyspnoea, fatigue,
angina, syncope on exertion, and ankle swelling, a raised jugular
venous pressure, right ventricular hypertrophy and an accentuated
pulmonary 2nd sound. The chest X-ray shows a large pulmonary
artery and ischaemic peripheral lung fields.

SILENT PULMONARY EMBOLISM

A rise of resting pulse rate, onset of atrial fibrillation, slight pyrexia
or the appearance of unexplained heart failure in a bed-ridden
patient may be the only evidence that pulmonary embolism has
occurred.

Prognosis

MASSIVE EMBOLISM

One third of patients die, 10% within ten minutes, 30% in one
hour and 60% in the new few hours or days. In the patients who
recover, return to normality is complete in young patients but
over the age of 40 some dyspnoea and right ventricular strain may
persist.

PULMONARY INFARCTION
Risk of a second pulmonary embolus in 25%.

MULTIPLE PERIPHERAL EMBOLISM
Death usually occurs from right ventricular failure within 2–5 years of the onset of symptoms.

Treatment
Prophylaxis involves prevention of all the factors outlined under aetiology but in spite of considerable efforts in this respect little reduction in the overall incidence of embolism seems to occur.

MASSIVE PULMONARY EMBOLISM
1   Oxygen and isoprenaline drugs for hypotension.
2   Anticoagulation and streptokinase.
    Heparin 12,500 units intravenously four hourly for two days, with phenindione or warfarin in appropriate doses to continue anti-coagulation subsequently. Streptokinase or urokinase is given intra-venously to lyse clot in lungs and leg veins.
3   Pulmonary embolectomy.
Indications—Persistent hypotension; episode of cardiac arrest.
Technique—Cardiopulmonary bypass is established through a median sternotomy, the pulmonary artery is opened and the thrombus is removed with manual squeezing of the lungs to remove peripheral emboli.
Results—If the patient's heart is beating when he reaches the operating theatre there is a reasonable chance of a successful outcome.

PULMONARY INFARCTION
1   Relief of pain.
2   Anticoagulation—Reduces the risk of recurrent embolism by 50%.
3   Vein ligation—Inferior vena caval or superficial femoral vein ligation is used if embolism recurs despite effective anticoagulation. The exact sites of ligation are determined by venography of both lower limbs. Plication operations leaving a small lumen in the cava have been recommended as alternatives to caval ligation.

MULTIPLE PERIPHERAL EMBOLISM
Long term anticoagulation to minimize further embolism. Treatment of established right ventricular failure, when it appears, with digitalis and diuretics.

Fat Embolism

Aetiology and pathology

Fat embolism may occur after bone fractures, external cardiac massage, or injection of therapeutic and diagnostic oils. Increased capillary permeability and congestion of the lungs is the effect of multiple fat globules in the pulmonary capillaries.

Clinical presentation

1   Sudden dyspnoea and chest pain with many crepitations over the lungs (systemic venous fat emboli carried to the lungs).
2   Coma or disorientation (cerebral fat embolism).
3   Petechial rash (emboli in the skin).
4   Haematuria.

Treatment

Oxygen and vasopressor drugs for hypotension.

Air Embolism

Aetiology and pathology

Inadvertent injection of air intravenously (15 ml/kg is the minimum necessary for production of symptoms) or opening a neck or cerebral vein. An air lock is caused in the right ventricular outflow tract and obstructs the circulation.

Clinical presentation

Features similar to massive pulmonary embolism but with a churning murmur over the right ventricle produced by the air lock.

Treatment

The patient is nursed with the right side and feet uppermost to keep the air out of the right ventricular outflow tract.

Foreign Body Embolism

Occasionally foreign bodies such as bullets enter a vein and are carried to the lungs. They can be removed at thoracotomy.

Carcinomatous Embolism

Carcinomatous tissue, particularly from breast and stomach, may produce subacute pulmonary embolism.

(e) PULMONARY HYPERTENSION

The normal systolic pressure in the pulmonary artery does not exceed 30 mm Hg and pulmonary hypertension is said to be present when the pulmonary arterial pressure is higher than this. Pressures of 100 mm Hg or more are not unusual in severe pulmonary hypertension.

Aetiology

Passive pulmonary hypertension
The pressure in the pulmonary artery must exceed the pulmonary venous pressure if blood is to flow through the lungs into the pulmonary veins, and any elevation of pulmonary venous pressure is necessarily accompanied by a rise in pulmonary artery pressure. Diseases causing a rise of pulmonary venous pressure (mitral stenosis, mitral incompetence, left ventricular failure) produce an equivalent rise in pulmonary artery pressure.

Reactive pulmonary hypertension
Some patients develop an active pulmonary arteriolar vasoconstriction as a reaction to a high pulmonary venous pressure. This greatly increases the resistance to blood flow through the lungs and the pressure in the pulmonary artery becomes disproportionately high. The precise mechanism initiating reactive pulmonary arterial vasoconstriction is unknown, but if the pulmonary hypertension is severe it has a profound influence on the course of the original disease. Twenty-five per cent of patients with severe mitral stenosis react in this way, but the proportion of patients with pure mitral incompetence or left ventricular failure doing so is smaller.

High pulmonary blood flow
Moderate increases of pulmonary blood flow can be accommodated without a rise in pulmonary artery pressure by dilatation of pulmonary blood vessels and opening up of previously closed channels. Large pulmonary blood flows (more than three times the normal) require an increased pulmonary pressure to maintain the flow. In the occasional patient the Eisenmenger reaction occurs (p. 85).

Reduction of pulmonary vascular bed
When two-thirds or more of the pulmonary vascular bed has been obliterated, an increase in pulmonary arterial pressure is necessary in order to maintain an adequate blood flow through the reduced vascular bed.

D

Diseases causing a reduction of the pulmonary vascular bed are:
1 Recurrent pulmonary emboli blocking many pulmonary arteries and arterioles. Emboli may be showers of blood clot from the leg veins or pelvic veins, tumour particles, bilharzia ova, or fat globules.
2 Widespread lung disease—emphysema, extensive pulmonary fibrosis.
3 Jugular venous pressure—large *a* wave 5 cms or more above the obliteration of the pulmonary arterial system takes place in childhood or early adult life without there being any evidence of the above factors.

Pathology of Pulmonary Hypertension

1 Pulmonary arterioles show hypertrophy of the media and thickening of the intima. In some the lumen is occluded and is by-passed by new thin-walled vessels.
2 The main pulmonary artery and larger branches are dilated (increased pressure). Pulmonary valve incompetence is usual when the pulmonary valve ring is involved in the pulmonary arterial dilatation.
3 The right ventricle is hypertrophied, and it dilates when right ventricular failure supervenes. Involvement of the tricuspid valve ring in this dilatation explains the frequent finding of tricuspid incompetence. The right atrium is hypertrophied due to the increased force necessary to fill the thickened right ventricle.

Clinical Presentation

Pulmonary hypertension reduces the cardiac output by imposing an abnormal load on the right ventricle, and eventually causes right ventricular failure.

Symptoms
Fatigue, breathlessness, angina pectoris, syncope (low cardiac output).
Oedema in later stages (right ventricular failure).
Haemoptysis (pulmonary infarction or rupture of abnormal blood vessels in lungs).

Clinical examination
1 General—cold extremities, peripheral cyanosis (low output).
2 Pulse—small amplitude (low output).
3 Jugular venous pressure—large *a* wave 5 cms or more above the sternal angle (forceful right atrial contraction).

4 Cardiac impulses—powerful heave to left of the sternum (right ventricular hypertophy). Palpable pulmonary valve closure (raised pulmonary artery pressure closing the valve forcibly).
5 Auscultation.
Pulmonary ejection click; soft pulmonary ejection murmur (dilated main pulmonary artery).
Very loud pulmonary second sound; blowing diastolic murmur at left sternal edge (pulmonary valve incompetence).
Pansystolic murmur in tricuspid area (functional tricuspid incompetence).
Atrial gallop in tricuspid area (increased forcefulness of right atrial contraction).

Electrocardiogram
Right ventricular hypertrophy and P pulmonale (right atrial hypertrophy).

Chest X-ray
Large pulmonary artery and main branches. Attenuated peripheral lung markings (obstructed and constricted peripheral arteries).

Increased transverse diameter of heart (enlarged right atrium and right ventricle).

Diagnosis of Underlying Cause of Pulmonary Hypertension

The complete diagnosis in severe pulmonary hypertension requires the discovery of the lesion initiating the reaction. This may be difficult, as the signs of pulmonary hypertension tend to obscure the signs of the original disease.

Mitral stenosis
Although the characteristic diastolic murmur may be inaudible (low cardiac output causing diminished flow through the mitral valve), the following features suggest the diagnosis:
1 Opening snap.
2 P mitrale on the electrocardiogram.
3 Chest X-ray: enlargement of the left atrium, the presence of calcium in the mitral valve or Kerley's lines at the bases.

Eisenmenger reaction
This term is used for the severe pulmonary hypertension occasionally found in association with intracardiac shunts and is reserved for those in whom blood flow is from right to left across the defect because of

the pulmonary hypertension. The presence of central cyanosis and finger clubbing indicates the right to left shunt, and suggests the diagnosis of Eisenmenger reaction. Identification of the site of the defect responsible for the shunt requires further investigation (p. 61).

Lung disease

Lung disease, such as chronic bronchitis and emphysema or diffuse interstitial fibrosis, is usually detected from the physical signs in the lungs and the chest X-ray.

Recurrent pulmonary embolism (thrombo-embolic pulmonary hypertension)

The symptoms commonly develop soon after childbirth, but the occurrence of pulmonary hypertension following an accident, a surgical operation or phlebothrombosis of the leg veins also make this diagnosis probable. There is not always a history of frank pulmonary embolism or infarction, nor does the chest X-ray provide evidence of infarction.

Prognosis

Severe pulmonary hypertension seriously limits the cardiac output, restricting the capacity for physical exertion. Disability and death are due to complications:

1   Right ventricular failure (prolonged strain on right ventricle).
2   Pulmonary embolism and infarction (slow circulation encourages thrombus formation in systemic veins).
3   Systemic embolism and brain abscess in the Eisenmenger groups (venous emboli can cross the defect into the systemic arterial system).
4   Massive haemoptysis (severe intra-pulmonary bleeding from a ruptured high pressure abnormal pulmonary vessel).

Treatment

Depends on the underlying cause of the hypertension.

Mitral valve disease

Can be remedied by mitral valvotomy or valve replacement. The presence of pulmonary hypertension considerably increases the immediate operative mortality but the long term results in survivors are good, because the pulmonary hypertension resolves when the left atrial pressure is lowered. Pulmonary and systemic embolism is particularly common in this group and anticoagulant therapy prior to surgery is recommended.

Eisenmenger Group
These patients have an average life expectancy of 30 or more years. Closure of the defect has no beneficial effect on the pulmonary hypertension and carries a prohibitively high operative mortality. Restriction of physical activities, with the use of digitalis and diuretics when arrhythmias and cardiac failure eventually appear, is all that can be offered.

Lung disease
Oxygen, bronchodilators, and antibiotics for respiratory infections are of value in reducing the pulmonary artery pressure when this is elevated because of lung disease. Extreme pulmonary hypertension is not usual in this group.

Thrombo-embolic pulmonary hypertension
Bed rest and anticoagulant therapy offer the best chance of keeping the pulmonary arterial pressure down and preventing further embolism to the lungs. If these measures are instituted early a cure may result. The fully developed case responds poorly to any form of therapy.

(f) DISORDERS OF CARDIAC RHYTHM

Sinus Rhythm

Normal sinus rhythm
The conducting system of the heart consists of specialized cells which exhibit a capacity for rhythmic spontaneous depolarization. The cells situated in the sino-atrial node have the fastest inherent rhythmicity, so that the sino-atrial node acts as the pacemaker of the heart by initiating the wave of depolarization which spreads across the atria to the atrio-ventricular node. From the atrio-ventricular node the impulse enters the bundle of His and reaches the ventricles through the right and left bundle branches and the Purkinje fibres. The sino-atrial node is under parasympathetic and sympathetic control, as is the atrio-ventricular node to a lesser extent. Depression of impulse formation in the sino-atrial node leads to the pacemaker function being taken over by cells further down the conducting system at a slower inherent rate. The normal heart rate is 120 per min in infancy and around 70–80 per min in adults.

Sinus arrhythmia

The heart rate speeds up during inspiration and slows during expiration. The complete reflex pathways by which respiration effects the sino-atrial node discharge rate are not known. Sinus arrhythmia is a normal finding, being particularly marked in the young and in people with high vagal tone.

Sinus arrhythmia is absent in atrial septal defects when the pulmonary blood flow is large.

Sinus tachycardia

A heart rate over 100 per min remaining under the control of the sino-atrial node. Causes include exertion, emotion, thyrotoxicosis, cardiac failure, blood loss and fever.

Sinus bradycardia

A heart rate under 60 per min remaining under the control of the sino-atrial node. Causes include: high vagal tone (such as in trained athletes), myxoedema, increased intra-cranial pressure, obstructive jaundice (bile salt action on sino-atrial node).

The Arrhythmias

An arrhythmia is present when the impulse initiating the contraction arises outside the sino-atrial node. The arrhythmias are classified according to the site of the cardiac pacemaker.

Supra-ventricular arrhythmias

(Pacemaker in the atria or the A–V node.)
Atrial or nodal extrasystoles, paroxysmal atrial or nodal tachycardia, atrial flutter, atrial fibrillation.

ATRIAL EXTRASYSTOLES AND NODAL EXTRASYSTOLES

A focus somewhere in the atria or in the A–V node discharges before the sino-atrial node, and initiates an impulse which spreads across the atria and down into the ventricles to cause a premature cardiac contraction. The sino-atrial node is discharged by this premature impulse and the next sinus impulse is delayed until the sino-atrial node has had time to recharge.

The regularity of the pulse is interrupted by a beat occurring earlier than normal.

Significance

Occasional extrasystoles are common in healthy people. Frequent extrasystoles may be the prelude to atrial fibrillation.

Electrocardiogram

The P wave of the extrasystole is deformed since the impulse spreads in an abnormal direction across the atria, having arisen in an abnormal site (Fig. 2.1(x)). The extrasystole occurs prematurely, the QRS is normal unless bundle branch block is present, and the pause after the extrasystole is not fully compensatory, i.e. the distance between the normal sinus beats is less than twice the basic cycle length.

Treatment

No treatment is required when atrial extrasystoles are an incidental finding. Frequent distressing palpitations can be diminished by the avoidance of factors known to precipitate extrasystoles—coffee, tea, alcohol and nicotine. Occasionally phenobarbitone, amytal or oral quinidine (200 mg t.d.s.) are necessary.

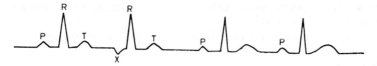

FIG. 2.1   Sinus rhythm with one atrial extrasystole 'x'

PAROXYSMAL ATRIAL AND NODAL TACHYCARDIA

The pacemaking function of the sino-atrial node is taken over by a rapidly discharging focus somewhere in the atria or the A–V node. There is a sudden onset of a fast regular heart rate over 150 per minute. The rate is completely regular and unchanging during the attack, but the patient may be able to halt the attack abruptly by some trick such as performing a Valsalva manœuvre, or by placing his head between his knees and holding his breath.

Significance

The heart is normal in at least 60% of patients. Attacks rarely last longer than a few hours and do not cause failure. The Wolff-Parkinson-White syndrome is responsible for some cases and should be suspected when the ventricular rate exceeds 200 per minute.

Electrocardiography

Normal QRS and T waves at a fast regular rate. Abnormally shaped P waves preceding each QRS complex are not always easily seen.

Treatment

Vagal stimulation either abruptly restores sinus rhythm by suppressing the abnormal pacemaking focus, or has no effect on the rhythm.

Methods of vagal stimulation are carotid sinus compression, eyeball compression, stimulation of vomiting reflex or injection of 1 mg prostigmine.

If vagal stimulation proves ineffective the ectopic focus may be suppressed by digitalization, oral quinidine or intravenous practolol. Direct current countershock can be expected to restore sinus rhythm in some 85% of cases and is indicated for prolonged attacks resistant to treatment.

ATRIAL FLUTTER

The atria are stimulated rapidly and regularly about 300 times per minute by an ectopic atrial pacemaker. The A–V node cannot conduct every impulse on to the ventricles, and the ventricles therefore beat at half or quarter of the atrial rate.

The pulse is usually regular and fast, and atrial flutter may be transient or persist for months. Vagal stimulation by carotid sinus pressure increases the degree of atrio-ventricular block, abruptly slowing the ventricular rate during the period of pressure only.

Significance

Ninety per cent of cases have underlying heart disease (rheumatic, ischaemic, hypertensive or congenital—particularly atrial septal defect). The fast ventricular rate is uncomfortable and may precipitate cardiac failure.

Electrocardiography

Rapid repetitive atrial stimulation from a single focus results in F waves on the electrocardiogram, all of identical shape and completely regular. The F waves are usually most prominent in lead II, giving the base line of the electrocardiogram a *picket fence* appearance (Fig. 2.2).

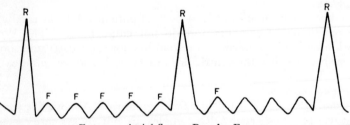

FIG. 2.2   Atrial flutter. Regular F waves

Treatment

1   Drugs. Digoxin 0·5 mg orally followed every 6 hours by 0·25 mg until impulse transmission through the A–V node and bundle of His

has been decreased to about 80 per min. Digitalization commonly converts the arrhythmia into atrial fibrillation and sinus rhythm may return on stopping the drug. If this fails oral quinidine may restore sinus rhythm when given to a patient who is adequately digitalized.
2   Synchronized direct current counter-shock is almost always effective in abolishing atrial flutter and is the treatment of choice.

ATRIAL FIBRILLATION

Small areas of the atrial muscle are stimulated at different moments and the atria have no co-ordinated contractions. Although there are approximately 600 stimuli per minute acting on the atria, ineffective irregular contractions of small areas of the atrial muscle result and only a proportion of these impulses are conducted through the A–V node to the ventricle.

The ventricular rate is fast and completely irregular.

Aetiology

Underlying disease   In most cases there is heart disease present, particularly common being rheumatic mitral valve disease, thyrotoxic heart disease and ischaemic heart disease. Less commonly other diseases are responsible for atrial fibrillation, such as atrial septal defect, cardiomyopathy and chronic lung disease. Occasionally atrial fibrillation follows thoracotomy, electrocution or an acute viral infection.

No underlying disease (lone atrial fibrillation)   Atrial fibrillation appearing in some adults for no discernable reason and compatible with a normal life span.

Factors favouring atrial fibrillation   Two factors are very important in determining the onset and the continuation of atrial fibrillation in any patient:
1   Advancing age.
2   Presence of a large atrium.

Effects of atrial fibrillation

Haemodynamic   Excessive heart rates on exertion are the rule despite adequate digitalization. The cardiac output does not rise normally on severe exertion but may be within normal limits at rest and during ordinary activities.

Systemic emboli   The incidence of systemic embolism is high in all types of atrial fibrillation, being highest in the rheumatic and the cardiomyopathy groups.

Electrocardiography

The abnormal atrial activity appears as small rapid irregular waves varying in size and shape. QRS complexes are of normal configuration but irregular in their rhythm (Fig. 2.3).

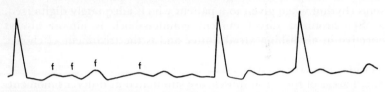

FIG. 2.3   Atrial fibrillation. Irregular fast 'f' waves. Irregular QRS complexes

Treatment

Slowing of ventricular rate   Digoxin is given until the ventricular rate is around 80 per min at rest. Digoxin decreases the number of impulses transmitted from the atria to the ventricles by its effect on the A–V node and bundle of His.

Long term anticoagulants   Indicated when the risk of systemic embolism is particularly high, e.g. atrial fibrillation with mitral stenosis.

Restoration of sinus rhythm

1   Usual indications.

(i) Thyrotoxic fibrillation persisting after control of thyrotoxicosis.

(ii) Rheumatic mitral stenosis in young patients after a successful valvotomy.

(iii) Atrial fibrillation precipitated by some factor no longer operating e.g. acute infection, thoracotomy.

2   Contra-indications. The factors originating the arrhythmia if still present will quickly defeat attempts to maintain sinus rhythm.

3   Methods.

(i) External direct current shock synchronized on the R wave of the electrocardiogram (p. 100).

(ii) Quinidine orally in increasing dosage until sinus rhythm is restored or until blood levels likely to cause toxic effects are approached. D.C. countershock is safer and is preferred.

Ventricular arrhythmias
(Pacemaker in the ventricles.)
Ventricular extrasystoles, ventricular tachycardia, ventricular fibrillation.

VENTRICULAR EXTRASYSTOLES
A focus in the ventricles is discharging early and takes over the pace-

making function of the sino-atrial node for one beat. The next sinus impulse finds the ventricles in a refractory state, and causes a pause following a ventricular extrasystole.

The regularity of the pulse is interrupted by a beat occurring earlier than normal.

Significance
Occasional ventricular extrasystoles can occur in a normal heart. Frequent ventricular extrasystoles indicate organic heart disease and may precede ventricular tachycardia or ventricular fibrillation.

Ventricular extrasystoles arising from more than one focus in the ventricles (multifocal ventricular extrasystoles) are particularly ominous.

Coupled ventricular extrasystoles, an extrasystole following every sinus beat, is often a sign of digitalis toxicity.

Electrocardiography (Fig. 2.4)
The QRS of the extrasystole is broadened and of abnormal shape, the exact configuration depending upon the site of the irritable focus. The distance between the normal QRS complexes flanking the ventricular extrasystole is exactly twice the normal cycle length i.e. the pause after the extrasystole is fully compensatory. Multifocal extrasystoles produce varying shapes of abnormal QRS complexes.

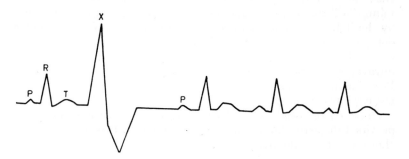

FIG. 2.4   Sinus rhythm with one ventricular extrasystole 'x'

Treatment
1   No treatment is required for an occasional extrasystole.
2   When they are due to digitalis toxicity the drug is discontinued and oral potassium is given.
3   Frequent extrasystoles thought to be precursors of more serious arrhythmias indicate the need for oral quinidine or intravenous lignocaine.

VENTRICULAR TACHYCARDIA

An irritable focus in the ventricle discharges rapidly and takes over the pacemaker function of the heart. These impulses are not usually conducted in a retrograde manner to the atria which therefore continue to beat at a normal rate under the sino-atrial node control.

The pulse rate is regular and rapid, usually 130/200 per minute.

Significance

Advanced disease of the ventricular muscle, usually ischaemic, or serious digitalis intoxication.

Electrocardiography

QRS complexes are bizarre and broad but identical one with another. P waves at a slower rate are identifiable bearing no fixed relationship to the QRS complexes.

Treatment

Drugs: Intravenous lignocaine Action—depresses ectopic foci. No significant effect on conduction, contractility, blood pressure or cardiac output.

Administration—begins with 50–100 mgs intravenously as a single bolus injection which has a rapid effect, persisting for 10–15 minutes (half life 10 minutes). Constant intravenous infusion of 2 mg per minute will maintain therapeutic blood level but must be preceded by the bolus injection. In heart failure or liver dysfunction, smaller doses are required for therapeutic blood levels.

Other drugs when lignocaine is not effective—Practolol 5–25 mgs intravenously, Sodium phenytoin 100–600 mgs intravenously, Procaine amide 100–800 mgs intravenously, Bretylium tosylate 0·1 mg/Kg intravenously.

Direct current countershock Very effective and carries little risk provided the arrhythmia is not digitalis induced. It is the method of choice for the acute arrhythmia.

VENTRICULAR FIBRILLATION

Depolarization of the ventricles is accomplished irregularly and patchily by rapid wandering impulses.

There is no co-ordinated contraction of the ventricles, no cardiac output and no peripheral pulse.

Aetiology

Often a terminal event after severe cardiac damage. Occasionally appears when underlying myocardial disease is not gross—myocardial infarction, aortic stenosis, complete heart block, electrocution or drug toxicity (adrenaline, digitalis, quinidine).

Electrocardiography
Completely irregular electrical activity of the fibrillating ventricles (Fig. 2.5).

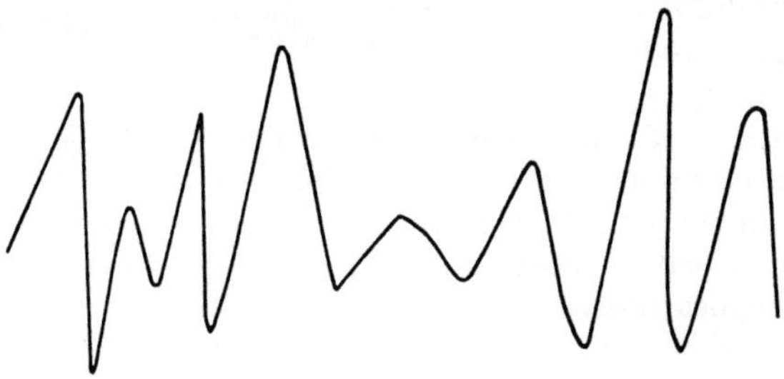

FIG. 2.5   Ventricular fibrillation

Treatment (see cardiac arrest, p. 102)
1   External cardiac massage.
2   Artificial ventilation.
3   Electrical defibrillation.
4   Drug therapy.

CAUSES OF A FAST REGULAR HEART RATE

Sinus tachycardia	Paroxysmal supra-ventricular tachycardia	Atrial flutter	Ventricular tachycardia
RATE			
Under 150 per min and varies slightly from hour to hour	150/200 per minute Does not vary	120/170 (2:1 A–V response) Does not vary unless A–V block changes	120/200 per minute Does not vary
CAROTID SINUS PRESSURE			
Slight slowing	Either abruptly restores sinus rhythm or does not affect heart rate	Abruptly slows the heart by increasing the degree of A–V block	No effect

An electrocardiogram taken when carotid sinus pressure is being exerted is valuable in the diagnosis of difficult cases, because slowing of the ventricular rate may unmask hidden atrial waves. The precise form of atrial arrhythmia can then be more easily seen.

Heart block

Atrio-ventricular heart block exists whenever there is delay or complete obstruction to the passage of the sino-atrial impulse to the ventricles.

AETIOLOGY

1   Degeneration and fibrosis of the atrio-ventricular bundle, cause unknown.

2   Ischaemic heart disease.

3   Depression of the conducting system by drugs (quinidine, digitalis, excess potassium), propranolol, procainamide.

4   Involvement of the bundle by chronic disease processes (syphilitic aortic disease, calcific aortic stenosis, ankylosing spondylitis).

5   Acute myocarditis.

  (i)   Acute rheumatic fever (first degree block usual).

  (ii)   Acute diphtheritic myocarditis (complete heart block, not permanent if patient survives).

6   Trauma to bundle during cardiac surgery.

7   Congenital heart block.

GRADES OF SEVERITY

First degree

Every atrial impulse is conducted to the ventricles after an abnormal delay in the conducting tissues. This is an electrocardiographic diagnosis (PR interval greater than 0·2 sec) the pulse remaining regular and at a normal rate.

Second degree

The bundle fails completely to conduct some impulses e.g. if only every second impulse is conducted there is a 2:1 atrio-ventricular block and the pulse rate is half the atrial rate.

Second degree heart block is subdivided into Mobitz Type I and Mobitz Type II heart block (Fig. 2.6).

Mobitz Type I   Block occurs high in A–V junction usually caused by a reversible condition such as inferior myocardial infarction or digitalis intoxication. Electrocardiogram shows Wenckebach phenomenon and normal QRS complexes. Progression to Stokes Adams attacks unusual.

Mobitz Type II   (Fig. 2.6) Block is in one bundle branch and dropped beats occur due to intermittent block in the other bundle branch, e.g. electrocardiogram shows right bundle branch block with left axis deviation and a normal PR interval (left axis deviation implies that the anterior division of the left bundle branch is blocked). Dropped beats occur without PR lengthening and without Wenckebach phenomenon when conduction ceases in the posterior division of the left bundle branch.

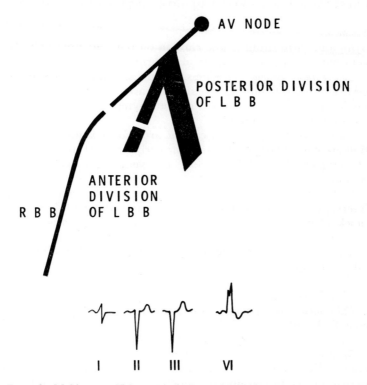

FIG. 2.6 Mobitz type II heart block. There is right bundle branch block shown on the electrocardiogram by an S wave in lead I and an R wave in VI. There is also interruption of the anterior division of the left bundle branch. This causes left axis deviation on the electrocardiogram. If the posterior division of the left bundle now fails to conduct sudden complete block will appear. The PR interval is not appreciably lengthened at any stage, before the appearance of complete block

Type II is a form of bilateral bundle branch block and usually progresses to complete block with slow bizarre QRS complexes and Stokes Adams attacks.

Third degree
Complete block. All atrial impulses are blocked in the conducting

system and the ventricular rate is controlled by a subsidiary pacemaker somewhere below the block (either in the A–V node or in the specialized conducting tissue of the ventricles).

CLINICAL PRESENTATION OF COMPLETE HEART BLOCK

Symptoms
Symptoms arise from a low cardiac output and from episodes of ventricular standstill or ventricular fibrillation.

Low cardiac output Tiredness, faintness, breathlessness and congestive cardiac failure appear if the heart rate is so slow that it is unable to maintain a normal output. Symptoms are inevitable at rates below 30 per minute.

Cardiac arrest Episodes of cardiac arrest or of ventricular fibrillation are particularly common in the early stages of the development of complete heart block before the ventricular pacemaker has become established.

Stokes Adams attacks (sudden transient loss of consciousness from interruption of cerebral blood flow) are most commonly seen in heart block. Convulsions occur in some patients during the attack and the resumption of the heart beat is accompanied by quick restoration of consciousness and a red flush in the skin as blood flows into anoxic dilated peripheral vessels.

Clinical Examination
Pulse and blood pressure Slow regular pulse of large amplitude. Systolic blood pressure is high and diastolic pressure low (large left ventricular stroke volume and peripheral vasodilatation).

Jugular venous pressure Irregular *cannon waves* whenever atrial contraction happens to coincide with ventricular systole—a large pressure wave travels into the superior vena cava and jugular veins because the tricuspid valve is closed during ventricular systole.

Auscultation Varying intensity of the first heart sound (varying degrees of separation of A–V valve cusps prior to ventricular systole because of the variable PR interval).

Electrocardiography
P waves normal in shape and rate. QRS complexes regular in rhythm but at a slow rate, the QRS complexes being normal if the ventricular pacemaker is in the A–V node or the bundle of His but wide and abnormal when the pacemaker is lower in the ventricles. The PR interval is completely variable from beat to beat, demonstrating the independence of the atria from the ventricles (Fig. 2.7).

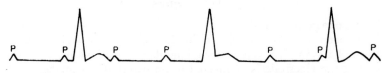

FIG. 2.7   Complete heart block. Completely variable PR interval

Chest X-ray
Large transverse diameter of heart (increased stroke volume is necessary to sustain the cardiac output at slow rates).

TREATMENT
If ventricular rate is over 40 beats per minute, the cardiac output is good, the QRS complexes are normal and there have been no Stokes Adams attacks, no specific therapy is necessary.
    Insertion of an electrical pacemaker is indicated for:
1   Stokes Adams attack.
2   Mobitz type II block (usually will progress to complete block with asystole).
3   Very slow ventricular rate with symptoms of low output or cardiac failure.

Drug therapy (occasionally useful)
Intravenous atropine may improve Mobitz type I block. Long acting preparation of isoprenaline hydrochloride (Saventrine 30–120 mg 4 hourly) will increase ventricular rate in chronic heart block but must be discontinued if ventricular extrasystoles are provoked. Steroids restore sinus rhythm in a few patients with acute inferior myocardial infarction (Mobitz type I).

ELECTRICAL PACEMAKING OF THE HEART

Indications

1   Stokes Adams attacks.
2   Slow ventricular rates unresponsive to medical treatment or intolerant of treatment.
3   Complete heart block in myocardial infarction if the cardiac output is poor and for all cases of Mobitz type II block.
4   Surgically induced complete heart block.
5   To drive the ventricles at a fast rate and thus prevent recurrent attacks of ventricular tachycardias—used when antiarrhythmic drugs have failed.

Techniques

Temporary pacemaker

A catheter electrode is placed in the apex of the right ventricle through a vein (arm vein, external jugular or subclavian). The other end of the electrode is connected to an external pacemaker which delivers 60–120 impulses per minute of 2–5 volts. A demand pacemaker is preferred—pacemaker senses the electrical activity of the ventricle and is inhibited if a spontaneous ventricular impulse occurs.

Permanent implanted pacemaker

As above but the small pacemaker is buried under the skin in the axilla or abdomen. Consistent pacing for three years can be expected before replacement becomes necessary. Implanted pacemakers may be of the fixed rate or demand type and may be connected to the heart by electrodes sewn on to the heart at thoracotomy if this is preferred.

EXTERNAL DIRECT CURRENT COUNTERSHOCK

An effective and safe method for the termination of many cardiac arrhythmias. A large electric current of short duration is passed through the chest and this depolarizes the heart, momentarily abolishing all electrical activity. Sinus rhythm is usually re-established as rhythmical electrical activity recommences.

Technique

1　Patient anaesthetized with thiopentone or diazepam.

2　Large electrodes placed on the skin overlying the heart, either at apex and base, or front and back of the chest.

3　One shock given at the peak of the R wave of the electrocardiogram (the shock is not given on the ascending limb of the T wave since this is the vulnerable period of the cardiac cycle and ventricular fibrillation can result. The apparatus automatically gives the shock at a predetermined point on the patient's electrocardiogram).

4　A shock of 40–400 J is necessary, depending on the nature of the arrhythmia and the build of the patient.

5　Usually digitalis is discontinued 36 hours prior to the shock as the technique is dangerous in the presence of excess digitalis.

6　Anticoagulants may be advisable for high embolic risk patients.

Indications

	Success rate
Atrial fibrillation (p. 91)	85%
Atrial flutter	Practically 100%
Paroxysmal atrial tachycardia not due to digitalis	80%
Ventricular tachycardia	95%
Ventricular fibrillation	Depends on aetiology

Contra-indications
Arrhythmias due to digitalis toxicity.

CARDIAC ARREST

Definition
Cardiac arrest is best defined as the cessation of an effective circulation due to:
1 Cardiac asystole.
2 Ventricular fibrillation.
3 Grossly inadequate cardiac output (extreme bradycardia or tachycardia, or feeble myocardial contractions).

Aetiology
Multiple factors are usually involved in any one case:

Myocardial anoxia

LOCAL
Coronary occlusion produces local anoxia of an area of myocardium surrounded by other areas which are properly oxygenated, a situation of electrical instability which readily precipitates ventricular fibrillation.

GENERAL
Any anoxic episode (anaesthesia with underventilation, airway obstruction etc.).

Reflex
Particularly vagal reflexes from tracheal stimulation (intubation,

inhaled vomit, tracheotomy) or traction on viscera at operation under light anaesthesia.

Drugs and electrolytes

1 Overdose of cardiac drugs—digitalis, quinidine, procaine amide.
2 Anaesthetic drugs—chloroform, cyclopropane, halothane, cocaine.
3 Electrolytes—high or low levels of potassium, high levels of calcium.

Other causes

Electrocution, drowning, air embolism.

Diagnosis of Cardiac Arrest

Sudden collapse accompanied by:
1 Unconsciousness.
2 Apnoea.
3 Absent pulses. Absent carotid pulsation is the best sign as the more peripheral vessels may be impalpable in any low cardiac output state.
4 Dilating pupils. The pupils start to dilate 30–45 seconds after circulatory arrest.

No further time is wasted in refinements of diagnosis such as electrocardiography, although this may be available if the patient is already connected to an ECG oscilloscope. Treatment is begun at once.

Treatment of Cardiac Arrest

Treatment may be divided into three stages: provision of an artificial circulation of oxygenated blood; restoration of a normal beat; and aftercare and treatment of complications.

Provision of an artificial circulation of oxygenated blood

Such provision entails external cardiac massage and artificial ventilation.

EXTERNAL CARDIAC MASSAGE

The patient is laid flat on a firm surface (floor or board) and the lower half of the sternum firmly but quickly depressed by the palms of the hands $1\frac{1}{2}$–2 inches in an adult (less for children) 80 times a minute.

The heart is compressed between the sternum and the vertebral column and its contained blood ejected into the pulmonary artery and aorta. Pressure is only applied over the lower half of the sternum because force applied elsewhere fractures ribs or damages the liver and spleen. Efficient cardiac compression results in a pulse being felt in a major artery and the return of circulation to the brain results in the pupils shrinking to a normal size.

ARTIFICIAL VENTILATION
The upper airway is cleared, the head extended and the jaw pulled forward. Ventilation can be performed by:
1 Mouth to mouth breathing.
2 Brook airway—Similar to mouth to mouth breathing but using an airway for better fit.
3 Ambu bag—A self-inflating bag and facemask allowing ventilation without a gas supply.
4 Endotracheal tube.
    Adequate ventilation is assessed by expansion of the chest with each inflation and by the patient's colour becoming pink.

Restoration of normal beat
Effective massage and ventilation alone may restart the heart and in any case are continued until a normal beat is restored.

DETERMINATION OF RHYTHM
An electrocardiograph is connected to the patient to diagnose whether the arrest is due to asystole, ventricular fibrillation or other rhythm disturbances.

INJECTION OF DRUGS
Sodium bicarbonate (80 mEq every 15 min of arrest) is given to counteract inevitable metabolic acidosis. Adrenaline (10 ml of 1:10,000) and calcium chloride (10 ml of 2% hydrated solution) increase the tone of the heart. Vasopressor drugs sustain the blood pressure once the heart has restarted. Lignocaine 1% and potassium chloride (40 mEq) depress myocardial irritability if relapse into ventricular fibrillation occurs.
    The drugs may be given into distended jugular veins, into an intravenous infusion or by direct intracardiac injection.

ELECTRICAL DEFIBRILLATION
Ventricular fibrillation is restored to normal rhythm by a shock from a D.C. defibrillator. One electrode is placed on the chest in the region of the cardiac apex and the other below the angle of the left scapula. A shock of 200 J is usually sufficient to halt ventricular fibrillation.

Aftercare and treatment of complications

AFTERCARE
1   Monitor pulse and blood pressure.
2   Oxygen by facemask.
3   Oscilloscope for cardiac rhythm.
4   Nasogastric tube to prevent inhalation of vomit.
5   Urinary catheter to recognize anuria early.

TREATMENT OF COMPLICATIONS

Renal failure
Acute cortical necrosis and anuria may occur and are treated with
large doses of frusemide, fluid restriction, ion exchange resins and if
necessary peritoneal dialysis.

Cerebral damage
Severe cerebral damage requires steroid therapy (e.g. dexametha-
sone for 8 days).

Respiratory failure
Assessed from arterial blood gas analysis. Mechanical ventilation is
used until spontaneous respiration is again adequate.

CHAPTER 3
TREATMENT OF HEART FAILURE

The principles of treatment of heart failure are:
1 Reduction of cardiac work.
2 Strengthening of myocardial contraction.
3 Removal of excess sodium and water and prevention of their re-accumulation.
4 Treatment of the cause of the failure.

Reduction of the Work Load on the Heart

Substantial reduction of the cardiac work load can be achieved by reducing the activity and therefore the oxygen requirements of the body.

Simple measures reducing body oxygen uptake
1 Bed rest. At least 3 weeks complete bed rest is advisable from the onset of heart failure. The cardiac output can be further reduced by having the patient supported on pillows at an angle of 45 degrees and lowering the legs.
2 Mental rest. Anxiety or excitement increases the cardiac output and cardiac work. Every effort is made to obtain mental relaxation and adequate sleep, with barbiturates or opiates if necessary.
3 Diet. Small light meals require less effort than large meals for their absorption.
4 Obvious abnormalities increasing the cardiac output, such as anaemia, are corrected.

Strengthening of Myocardial Contraction
Digitalis
Digitalis increases the contractility of the failing heart and is indicated for all patients in cardiac failure. Digitalis is taken up by heart muscle and also to a lesser extent by somatic muscle and the liver, and the aim of therapy is to build up the concentration of digitalis in the heart until maximum benefit is obtained and thereafter to replace the daily loss with a smaller maintenance dose. The dosage required to achieve these aims varies from patient to patient, and the optimum dosage is only slightly below the toxic level. In

heart muscle digitalis shares specific receptor sites on the cell membrane with potassium, and binding of digitalis at these sites is high if the potassium level is low.

ACTIONS OF DIGITALIS

1 Inotropic effect. A direct action on the heart increasing the force of cardiac contraction.

2 Chronotropic effects.

(i) Conduction velocity. Increased in the atria and ventricles. Slowed in the atrioventricular junction both by direct effect and by a reflex vagal action.

(ii) Refractory period. Increased in the atrioventricular junction. Shortened in the ventricles.

3 Automaticity. Enhanced in ventricular Purkinje cells, atrioventricular junctional cells and atrial cells. Hence tendency to extrasystoles and tachycardia with overdosage.

4 Heart rate. Minimal direct effect. Slowing may occur from improvement in haemodynamics when given for heart failure and also through a vagal effect.

DIGITALIZING DOSE

Digoxin, usually the drug of choice, is well absorbed by mouth, not metabolized to any appreciable extent and renal excretion determines the duration and magnitude of its effect—in normal renal function the plasma half-life of digoxin is about 34 hours. An initial dose of 0·5 mg followed at 6 hourly intervals of 0·25 mg up to a total dose of 2–3 mg or until early signs of toxicity appear will produce digitalization. Intramuscular digoxin can be given when absorption from the alimentary tract is poor.

For rapid effect intravenous digoxin, maximum dosage 1 mg, will begin to act in 15 minutes and reach a maximal effect in 3 hours. Intravenous ouabain 0·3–0·6 mg acts within 5 minutes but the abrupt action of this drug makes it unsuitable for long term use. Intravenous digitalis preparations are not given to any patient already taking these drugs.

MAINTENANCE DOSAGE

Approximately 0·5 mg digoxin daily. Elimination from the body is by the kidney. Smaller maintenance dosage is required when the glomerular filtration rate is reduced.

JUDGMENT OF ADEQUATE DIGITALIZATION

Assessment of the adequacy of the therapy involves consideration of the total amount given together with careful enquiry for toxic effects.

The patient's sensitivity to digitalis is increased in:
Hypothyroidism.
Low serum potassium states, including diuretic therapy.
Old age. The kidneys excrete digoxin slowly.
Low serum magnesium.
High serum calcium.

The aim is to give a sufficient dosage to obtain the beneficial effects without any toxic symptoms and signs. Measurement of plasma levels of digoxin is useful in gastrointestinal disease, impaired renal function and in atrial fibrillation with a fast ventricular rate despite apparently adequate dosage.

CHOICE OF PREPARATION

Digoxin is usually the drug of choice. Available as tablets 0·25 mg and 0·0625 mg, as a paediatric elixir 0·05 mg per ml and in solution for intramuscular and intravenous injection.

Digitoxin. 0·1 mg tablet approximately equivalent to 0·25 mg digoxin. 70% metabolized in the liver, 30% excreted by the kidney. Half life in the body is 6 days. Provides a smooth level but is a much less flexible drug than digoxin.

TOXIC EFFECTS

Anorexia, malaise, headache, nausea, vomiting.
Digitalis induced rhythm disturbances:
Coupled ventricular extrasystoles, sinus arrest, heart block of all degrees, paroxysmal atrial tachycardia with block, ventricular tachycardia and ventricular fibrillation.

If toxic symptoms occur it is usually sufficient to withhold the drug for one or two days and it can then be restarted at a reduced maintenance dose. Serious poisoning demands the immediate withdrawal of the drug and the correction of any potassium depletion. For established serious arrhythmias intravenous lignocaine or phenytoin are often effective. Beta-adrenergic blocking drugs are also effective but must usually be avoided because heart failure may be precipitated.

Removal of Excess Sodium and Water

Many of the symptoms of heart failure can be attributed to an excess of sodium and water:
Breathlessness from fluid in the interstitial tissues of the lungs.
Abdominal distension and pain from an enlarged liver and an engorged gut.
Ankle swelling due to excess of fluid in the interstitial tissues.

A wide variety of diuretics are available which cause the kidneys to excrete sodium and water:

Oral diuretics

DOSAGE

Oral diuretics are given daily until the patient has lost the excess sodium, following which the dosage is adjusted to maintain this state. Where possible diuretic therapy should be intermittent, allowing some days between courses, as side effects from electrolyte imbalance are then less frequent.

The wide range of diuretics available include:
Chlorothiazide (0·5 G–2·0 G daily).
Hydrochlorothiazide (50–200 mg daily).
Bendrofluazide (5–20 mg daily).
Frusemide (40 mg tablets).
Ethacrynic acid (50 mg tablets).

CHOICE OF DIURETIC

Using the first three, sodium excretion increases with increasing dosage only to a certain level, after which further increase in diuretic therapy has no demonstrable effect. Frusemide and ethacrynic acid may be increased progressively with increasing diuretic effect.

Frusemide is the drug of choice for severe heart failure and has a short duration of action, the diuresis being almost completed within 2 hours of oral administration. A dosage of 40 mg twice daily is usual but may be increased greatly. Ethacrynic acid can be combined for a more powerful effect.

The less powerful diuretic action of bendrofluazide is more prolonged and is preferred when the acute situation is under control.

POTASSIUM SUPPLEMENTS

Potassium supplements are necessary to make good the potassium loss caused by these diuretics, whenever diuretics are given daily or on alternate days. Tablets containing potassium salts, including tablets in which potassium is combined with the diuretic, can cause small bowel ulceration with bleeding and eventual stenosis of the bowel. The best way to give potassium is in the form of effervescent potassium tablets, two tablets thrice daily, or as slow release potassium tablets 600 mg four times daily. The latter also supplies chloride ions and is preferable on this account.

1 Increased potassium loss. This may precipitate digitalis toxicity in digitalized patients. Potassium depletion also causes weakness, muscle cramps, and postural hypotension.
2 Decreased glucose tolerance, aggravating diabetes or any diabetic tendency.
3 Uraemia is precipitated in the presence of poor renal function. The glomerular filtration rate is decreased by the oral diuretics.
4 Gout is provoked in some patients. Oral diuretics increase the uric acid in the tissues and the blood.

Aldosterone antagonists
Spironolactone (25 mg–50 mg q.d.s.) antagonizes the action of aldosterone but is of limited value in cardiac failure, since aldosterone levels are not always high. Indications include:
1 Low potassium state or a tendency to this despite the addition of potassium supplements. Spironolactone reduces the renal excretion of potassium and is a useful supplement to the oral diuretic regime in these patients.
2 Oedema resistant to oral diuretics of the thiazide group occasionally responds when spironolactone is added.

Removal of the Cause of the Failure

Effective treatment of the cause of heart failure offers the best prospect of cure e.g. successful abolition of cardiac arrhythmias, cure of thyrotoxicosis, control of systemic hypertension, correction of anaemia, treatment of alcoholism and nutritional deficiencies, cardiac surgery to correct valve lesions or congenital cardiac defects. Adequate medical treatment prior to surgery will improve the results.

Specific Forms of Failure

Acute pulmonary oedema due to left ventricular failure

POSTURE
The pulmonary venous pressure is promptly lowered by placing the patient upright in bed or on a chair with his legs down over the side.

DRUGS
Morphine (10 mg intravenously) reduces anxiety, dilates the systemic veins and lowers the systemic blood pressure.
Aminophylline (500 mg intravenously slowly) releases any

bronchospasm, improves renal blood flow and may improve myocardial function.

Frusemide (20 mg intravenously) rapidly initiates a renal diuresis of sodium and water.

Digoxin. An initial dose of 1 mg is given intramuscularly to a patient not already receiving digitalis.

OXYGEN

Supplied by face mask partially corrects the hypoxaemia caused by acute pulmonary oedema.

SPECIAL MEASURES

Tourniquets applied to the lower limbs, sufficiently tightly to obstruct venous return from the limbs, effectively removes blood temporarily from the circulation. Alternatively one pint can be removed by venesection, but this will produce a temporary anaemia and is avoided unless the situation cannot be controlled by other means.

Intermittent positive pressure respiration is very effective in controlling pulmonary oedema. If this is required for more than seven days a tracheostomy must be performed. This method of treatment is reserved for those in whom there is the probability that the acute pulmonary oedema is a temporary incident.

Heart failure in infancy

POSTURE

The infant is nursed at an angle of 45 degrees with the head raised, and this position is maintained by lengths of adhesive strapping applied along the back or by a pad under the buttocks.

FEEDING

A thin polythene naso-gastric tube is passed for feeding, to remove the work of sucking, and the milk given is sodium free.

DIGITALIS

Digitalizing dose: 0·04 mg per kg body weight. Half of this is given at once, followed by a quarter eight hours later and the final quarter in a further eight hours.

Maintenance dose: 0·01 mg per kg of body weight per day.

DIURETICS

Frusemide 1 mg per kg body weight intramuscularly.

Chlorothiazide 20 mg per kg body weight on alternate days along with potassium chloride 50 mg per kg body weight.

CONTINUOUS OXYGEN

Supplied by an oxygen tent or incubator, aiming to raise the oxygen content of the inspired air to about 40%.

SEDATION

One of the following drugs is usually given to prevent restlessness and the increase in heart work which results.

Morphine 0·1 mg per kg body weight every six to eight hours.

Pethidine 1 mg per kg body weight every six to eight hours.

Phenobarbitone 3 mg per kg body weight every eight hours.

CHAPTER 4
SURGERY IN HEART DISEASE

The ultimate success of any cardiac operation depends as much on meticulous preoperative study and treatment of the patient, followed by intensive care after surgery, as on technical correction of the defect.

Indications for Surgery in Heart Disease

The presence of a technically correctable cardiac lesion is an indication for surgery if:
1 Medical treatment fails to relieve symptoms. The severity of symptoms that demand operation depends on the risks of the corrective procedure, e.g. mitral valvotomy is recommended for mild symptoms but symptoms have to be relatively severe before multiple valve replacement is recommended today because of its long term complications.
2 The current mortality and morbidity of surgery are less than that of the natural history of the lesion. For instance, a symptomless persistent ductus arteriosus is an indication for surgery because of the low risk of the operation and the higher risk of bacterial endarteritis without surgery.

Contra-indications to Surgery

Even though the above indications apply, operation is not recommended if the situation is physiologically irrecoverable due to long-standing changes in the heart and circulation:
1 Irreparable damage to the myocardium, e.g. extensive myocardial infarction.
2 Pulmonary vascular resistance at systemic level. Closure of septal defects in the Eisenmenger situation (p. 87) is uniformly fatal.
3 Irreversible damage to other systems e.g. liver, lungs, kidneys. Despite correction of the cardiac lesion, death will occur from hepatic, respiratory and renal failure.

Physiological Disturbances Associated with Cardiac Surgery
Any operation on the heart produces temporary physiological deterioration during the post-operative period and a cardiac,

pulmonary, hepatic and renal reserve is necessary for survival however well the primary defect has been corrected.

Changes inherent in thoracotomy

A thoracic incision results in pain on breathing which in turn reduces
ventilation. The vital capacity falls and underventilated alveoli cause
a respiratory acidosis, ventilation/perfusion mismatch (see below)
and a fall in arterial oxygen tension.

Changes inherent in cardiotomy

Opening the pericardium does no harm unless a post-pericardiotomy
syndrome (p. 299) develops. An atrial incision also carries little
inherent morbidity unless it is carried too close to the S.A. node,
when arrhythmias may follow.

Right ventriculotomy for closure of ventricular septal defects
damages muscle fibres and limits the power of contraction, and right
bundle branch block develops. Adoption of a transverse rather than
a vertical ventriculotomy reduces this damage to a minimum by not
interfering with the synchrony of contraction of the ventricle.

Clamping the aorta for open operations on the aortic valve necessarily render the heart ischaemic and provision has to be made for perfusion of the coronary arteries with indwelling cannulae (Fig. 4.5).

Changes inherent in cardiopulmonary bypass

BLOOD DAMAGE

Haemolysis, denaturation of proteins, and microembolism with
particles of fibrin, fat, silicone, aggregated red cells and air bubbles
occur, the effects increasing with the length of bypass and amount of
suction of blood from heart and pericardium. Platelets are reduced
in number and clotting factors diluted. Fibrinolysis may be activated.
Later a normochromic normocytic anaemia is common.

ALTERATION OF PULMONARY FUNCTION

Patchy collapse of alveoli and increased stiffness of the lungs,
maximal on the second postoperative day, allows shunting of
pulmonary arterial blood through underventilated alveoli to the
pulmonary veins, so that the arterial blood may become desaturated
(ventilation/perfusion mismatch). The cause of this syndrome is
unknown. It is of particular importance in infant lungs and is
aggravated by a high left atrial pressure.

ELECTROLYTE DISTURBANCE

Loss of potassium ions in the urine is inevitable during and after cardiopulmonary bypass if a diuresis is produced by a perfusion primed with dextrose or mannitol. This may critically lower the level of potassium and cause dangerous arrhythmias.

ACID BASE CHANGES
With 'normal' flows of oxygenated blood, there is little anoxia of tissues but if the output of the machine falls or the blood is under-oxygenated, metabolic acidosis occurs which may depress myocardial contractility.

Preparation for Operation

For surgery to have its best chance of success the patient must reach the operating table with an accurate assessment of the underlying lesion and its complications, and in as good a circulatory condition as possible.

Accurate diagnosis
The site of the lesion, the presence of associated lesions and the severity of complicating factors such as pulmonary hypertension are elucidated before operation because diagnosis on the operating table is difficult, time-consuming and often incomplete.

General preparation of the patient
Psychological preparation of the patient and relatives is facilitated by explaining the operative and post-operative management, particularly if positive pressure ventilation is likely to be necessary. Anaemia is corrected and other coincident diseases e.g. diabetes, controlled.

Cardiac failure is corrected or reduced to a minimum by a suitable period of rest, diet and drugs. Electrolyte imbalance is corrected. Bronchospasm, bronchial secretions and infection are controlled by admission to hospital, antispasmodics, antibiotics, physiotherapy and stopping smoking.

General Operative Technique

Anaesthesia
Anoxia or hypotension are dangerous during anaesthesia, particularly when the pulmonary vascular resistance is raised or after pulmonary embolism. Anoxia increases this resistance and an already limited cardiac output may fall critically.

Access to the heart
A median sternotomy can be used for almost any operation, but is

especially valuable for operations on the ascending aorta, pulmonary artery, right ventricle and left atrium behind the right. A right anterolateral incision in the 4th or 5th intercostal space may be used for cosmetic reasons for operations on the right or left atrium. A similar incision on the left side can be used for operations on the mitral valve. A left posterolateral incision is used for access to the descending thoracic aorta and ductus arteriosus.

Access to the Defect

A few operations can be effectively performed by touch without being able to see the lesion (closed heart surgery) but the majority require such accurate technique that a direct view of the lesion is essential (open heart surgery).

Closed heart surgery
The circulation is maintained by the patient's heart throughout the operation which is carried out by touch rather than sight. The advantages of closed heart surgery are that it is cheap and simple, requiring only such equipment as valvotomes and dilators. Its disadvantages are inevitable inaccuracy and the limited number of possible operations because the lesion has to be correctable by crude techniques without obstructing the flow of blood through the heart for more than a few beats. Defects suitable for closed heart surgery are:
1 Mitral stenosis (dilated through left ventricle).
2 Pulmonary stenosis in Fallot's Tetralogy (dilated or punched out through the right ventricle).
3 Transposition of the great arteries (palliation by making an atrial septal defect if balloon atrioseptostomy fails).
4 Operations outside the chambers of the heart (shunt operations for Fallot's Tetralogy, pericardiectomy for constrictive pericarditis and operations on the aorta for persistent ductus arteriosus and coarctation).

Open heart surgery
The defect is corrected under direct vision by occluding the inflow of venous blood from the superior and inferior venae cavae, opening the heart and emptying it of blood. There is no cardiac output during this period so that the limiting factor of the technique is cerebral damage from ischaemia. The length of time available for surgery is prolonged by protecting the brain during the period of circulatory stasis or by maintaining a circulation artificially while the heart is excluded.

E

The variants of open heart surgery are inflow occlusion at normal temperatures, 30°C and 15°C, and the use of cardiopulmonary bypass. Only cardiopulmonary bypass is widely used for open heart surgery today but may be combined with moderate (30°C) or profound (15°C) hypothermia.

Profound hypothermia is particularly valuable in infancy when the time on cardiopulmonary bypass has to be kept to a minimum because of its effect on infant lung function. The temperature is reduced to 15°C and the circulation discontinued for an hour during the intracardiac procedure. Rapid rewarming then follows. Total correction procedures are now possible in infancy with this technique.

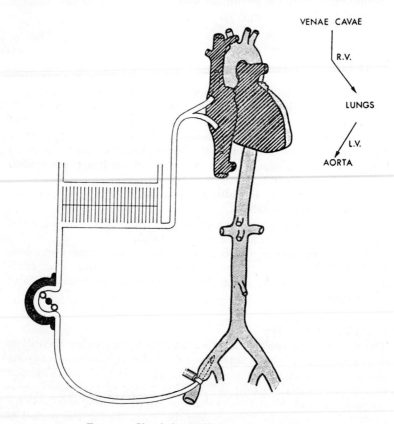

FIG. 4.1   Circuit for cardio-pulmonary bypass

Cardiopulmonary Bypass

Technique

The heart and lungs are excluded from the circulation, their function being taken over by a pump and an artificial oxygenator (Fig. 4.1). Venous blood is withdrawn by gravity through catheters in the superior and inferior venae cavae into the oxygenator from which it is pumped back into the aorta through the femoral artery—partial bypass (Fig. 4.2). When the cavae are snared tight around the catheters, all the venous return is diverted into the oxygenator—total bypass (Fig. 4.3). The heart may now be opened and is dry except for coronary and bronchial venous blood which is sucked out, defoamed and returned to the oxygenator (Fig. 4.4). Coronary arteries are separately perfused by indwelling catheters during operations on the aortic valve (Fig. 4.5). After closure of cardiotomies and exclusion of air, the caval snares are released (partial bypass) and finally bypass is discontinued (Fig. 4.1).

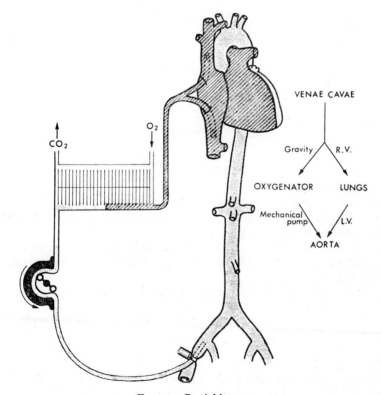

FIG. 4.2   Partial bypass

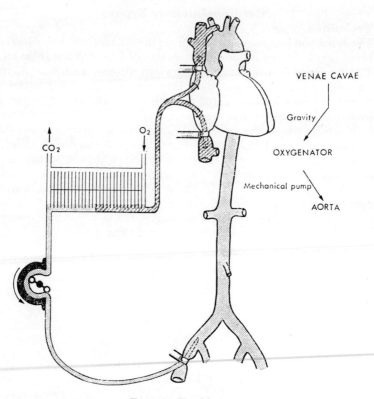

FIG. 4.3   Total bypass

Oxygenators

Venous blood may be oxygenated in three ways:

1   By bubbling oxygen through it and defoaming the froth with silicone (bubble oxygenators).

2   Making a thin film of blood in an atmosphere of oxygen on a screen which is either still or rotating (stationary screen and rotating disc oxygenators).

3   Separating blood from oxygen by a thin membrane (membrane oxygenators).

The oxygenator in most common use is the disposable plastic bubble oxygenator.

Profound hypothermia

The temperature of the patient is reduced to 15°C by passing the oxygenated blood through a heat exchanger. The circulation is discontinued for an hour. This technique is of value in infants to minimize lung damage from prolonged bypass and where there is a leak from aorta to the heart, e.g. persistent ductus arteriosus.

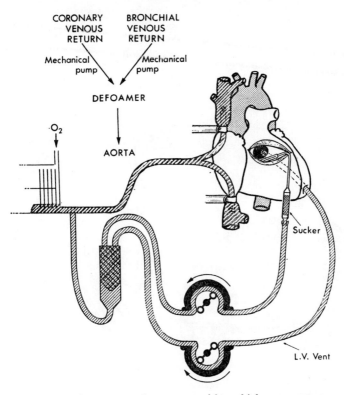

FIG. 4.4   Management of coronary and bronchial venous return

Postoperative Management

Maintenance of an adequate cardiac output is the object of post-operative management.

Cardiac output

The cardiac output is assessed directly or indirectly from evidence of perfusion of brain (cerebral function), kidneys (hourly urine output above 0·5 ml/kg/hr) and feet (warm, filled veins, palpable arterial pulses). The cardiac output depends on the stroke volume and heart rate. The stroke volume is adjusted by altering the filling pressure and myocardial contractility. The heart rate is maintained with drugs or a pacemaker. If the cardiac output remains low, the effects of poor tissue perfusion are minimized by protecting the kidneys and reducing the body's oxygen consumption.

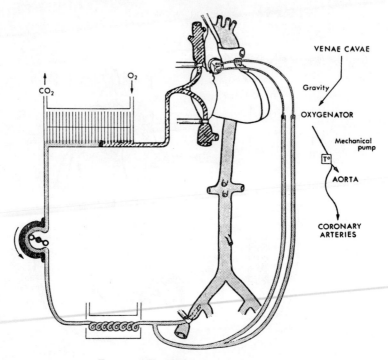

FIG. 4.5   Circuit for aortic valve surgery

STROKE VOLUME

Filling pressure of ventricles
The filling pressure (atrial pressure) of the ventricle most under stress, e.g. left ventricle in aortic and mitral disease, right ventricle in pulmonary stenosis, is raised by transfusion until the cardiac output is judged to be adequate. Further transfusion only causes pulmonary venous congestion (stiff lungs, falling PO_2) and systemic congestion (rising haemocrit). 15 mm Hg from sternal angle (25 mm Hg from LA level) is maximum.

Myocardial contractility
If the cardiac output is inadequate with high filling pressures, myocardial contractility can be improved by isoprenaline (Isuprel) or

adrenaline infusion, digoxin and calcium. Metabolic acidosis, which depresses contractility, is corrected if present with sodium bicarbonate. Arterial blood oxygenation is maintained by keeping the lungs clear of secretions and atelectasis and avoiding excessively high LA pressures.

HEART RATE
The heart rate is kept near 100/min with isoprenaline or a pacemaker (wires implanted at surgery). If necessary any arrhythmia is dealt with.

PREVENT EFFECTS OF REDUCED CARDIAC OUTPUT ON OTHER TISSUES
1 Maintain urine output (mannitol, frusemide). Kidney tolerates ischaemia better if producing urine.
2 Reduce oxygen consumption of body. Positive pressure ventilation, prevent hyperpyrexia, if necessary curarize.

Postoperative Complications of Cardiac Surgery

Low cardiac output
A low cardiac output may be due to one or more of six complications, all of which present with the signs of a low cardiac output (restlessness, cold venoconstricted extremities, peripheral cyanosis, sinus tachycardia, falling urinary output, low mixed venous oxygen saturation from increased tissue extraction, and metabolic acidosis in the arterial blood) plus their own characteristic diagnostic features.

HAEMORRHAGE
Haemorrhage is due to inadequate surgical haemostasis or decreased coagulability of the blood. In addition to the signs of a low cardiac output, the patient is pale and sweating, breathing rapidly, with a low venous pressure. Treatment involves transfusion of blood and correction of the cause of the haemorrhage by return of the patient to the theatre for proper haemostasis or by infusion of appropriate clotting factors.

TAMPONADE
Tamponade is due to haemorrhage into the pericardium preventing filling of the ventricles. It presents with a low cardiac output but with pulsus paradoxus and a raised jugular venous pressure with a dominant systolic descent. It is treated by immediate thoracotomy.

CARDIAC FAILURE

Cardiac failure may be due to myocardial damage or persistence or recurrence of defects. It presents with a low cardiac output, a raised jugular venous pressure with a dominant *y* descent, a third sound on auscultation and perhaps basal pulmonary crepitations. It is treated by oxygen, digitalis, isoprenaline, diuretics and if necessary removing the work of respiration by positive pressure ventilation.

Artificial maintenance of the circulation with intraortic balloons synchronized with the electrocardiogram, inflating during diastole and deflating during systole, has been shown to increase coronary and systemic perfusion. The artificial heart is at present a research project only, due to difficulties in maintaining the power source and to thrombosis in the 'heart'.

ARRHYTHMIAS

Arrhythmias are recognized by the pulse and electrocardiogram, and are corrected by D.C. countershock or drugs appropriate to the arrhythmias (pp. 88–95).

FLUID AND ELECTROLYTE IMBALANCE

Incorrect provision of water and sodium can give rise to an abnormally low blood volume. A low potassium level may lead to arrhythmias, particularly if digitalis is being used, and too high a potassium level to reduced myocardial contractility and asystole.

PULMONARY EMBOLISM

Massive pulmonary embolism presents as a low cardiac output associated with dyspnoea, some rise in jugular venous pressure and a change in the electrocardiogram to right ventricular strain. Treatment is anticoagulation, phlebography followed by appropriate vein ligation, or pulmonary embolectomy on cardiopulmonary bypass, depending on the urgency of the situation (p. 81).

Respiratory failure

Following a cardiac operation, the most common respiratory complication is patchy collapse of alveoli through which pulmonary arterial blood still flows. Such ventilation/perfusion mismatch produces a lowered arterial oxygen saturation which is detrimental to cardiac function. The collapse may be due to a high pulmonary venous pressure, sputum retention, hypoventilation or trauma in extracorporeal apparatus (*perfusion lung*). Correction involves reduction of the left atrial pressure, removal of secretions and encouragement of ventilation by physiotherapists, though positive pressure ventilation may be necessary in severe cases.

Renal failure

Oliguria following cardiac surgery is usually due to acute tubular necrosis caused by a low renal blood flow and pulse pressure. It is recognized by the passage of less than 400 ml per day of poorly concentrated urine in spite of large doses of frusemide (up to 500 mg). The blood urea and serum potassium rise. Treatment involves restriction of water intake to 400 ml daily and reduction of the serum potassium level with ion exchange resins. Peritoneal dialysis is used if conservative measures fail.

Hepatic failure

Jaundice is not uncommon after cardiac surgery, but hepatic failure is usually the late result of a low cardiac output and is often accompanied by renal failure. There is no effective treatment.

Cerebral damage

Cerebral damage is due to anoxia or embolism of air, thrombus, calcium, fat or silicone and may be complicated by cerebral oedema. Cerebral damage is treated by maintaining a normal blood pressure, a reduced carbon dioxide tension (30–35 mm Hg) with positive pressure ventilation, avoiding hyperpyrexia, and giving steroids (e.g. dexamethazone).

CHAPTER 5
CONGENITAL HEART DISEASE

GENERAL

Incidence

One case per 200 live births.

Aetiology

Environmental factors
The heart has reached its fully differentiated form by the end of the second month of gestation and thereafter is less susceptible to adverse influences. Factors known to cause congenital cardiac malformations, particularly if they operate during the first two months, are:
Maternal rubella and other virus diseases.
Thalidomide and possibly other drugs.
Radiation.
Hypoxia at confinement may cause persistent patency of the ductus arteriosus.

Hereditary influences
Genetic factors probably play only a minor part in determining congenital heart disease, and major chromosomal abnormalities are not usually present.

However some families do have a high incidence of congenital heart disease, the cardiac malformations being similar in the affected members of any one family.

Frequency of Specific Malformations

The following lesions are most commonly encountered in clinical practice:
Ventricular septal defect.
Atrial septal defect.
Persistent ductus arteriosus.
Fallot's tetralogy.
Pulmonary stenosis.

Coarctation of the aorta.

Transposition of the great vessels.

No figures are given for the relative frequency of these lesions as this largely depends on the age group under study.

Prevention

The risk of congenital heart disease can be substantially reduced by carefully shielding the pregnant woman from factors known to affect the foetus adversely.

Maternal rubella

Deliberate exposure of young girls before the reproductive age to rubella will give a lasting active immunity.

A viraemia can persist for some weeks after a rubella infection and it is recommended that conception be avoided for two months; otherwise there is a danger of infecting the foetus.

For mothers in contact with rubella in the early months of pregnancy, gamma globulin may offer some protection provided this is administered within ten days of the exposure to infection.

Thalidomide and other drugs

The prescription of any drugs to pregnant women should be kept to a minimum as no drug can be regarded as completely safe during early pregnancy.

Radiation

Routine radiography during pregnancy is avoided.

CHAPTER 6
RHEUMATIC FEVER

Aetiology

A small proportion of people infected with a Group A haemolytic streptococcus develop rheumatic fever. No specific type of Group A streptococcus is responsible, and the reason why some people respond to infection in this way is not known. Any infection by the Group A streptococcus can be responsible for rheumatic fever— throat infections and scarlatina are the two most common.

Rheumatic fever is uncommon before the age of 4 and after the age of 18, and both the incidence and the severity of the disease are at present decreasing in the Western world.

Pathology

The endocardium, the myocardium and the pericardium may all be affected.

Endocarditis. Acute inflammation, with the formation of Aschoff nodules during the acute illness. Chronic rheumatic heart disease represents the end result of inflammation and destruction of valve tissue (pp. 130, 141, 150, 159, 185, 187).

Myocarditis. Heart failure during the acute attack indicates severe involvement of the myocardium.

Pericarditis. When this is recognizable clinically the disease is usually severe.

Clinical Features

1   History of streptococcal infection 10–21 days previously.
2   Pyrexia, high erythrocyte sedimentation rate and anaemia then appear, accompanied by more than one of the following major manifestations of rheumatic fever:

(i) Polyarthritis—Pain, swelling, tenderness, heat and redness in the joints, migrating from one to another and involving primarily the knee, ankle, elbow, wrist and hand joints.

(ii) Carditis.
Endocarditis—Development of heart murmurs.
Myocarditis—Cardiac enlargement; congestive cardiac failure; prolonged PR interval on the E.C.G.

Pericarditis—Pericardial friction rub.

(iii) Subcutaneous nodules—Firm painless nodules appearing over the extensor surfaces of elbows, knees and wrists, over the occipital region and over the thoracic and lumbar spinous processes.

(iv) Erythema marginatum—Evanescent pink rash on trunk and proximal part of the extremities, never on the face. The erythematous areas have pale centres and serpiginous margins without induration. It is uncommon, but characteristic of rheumatic fever when present.

(v) Chorea—Purposeless involuntary rapid movements, associated with muscle weakness. This is a late manifestation of the rheumatic process, occurring more than two months after the streptococcal infection.

Laboratory Confirmation

Laboratory evidence of recent streptococcal infection can be obtained in almost all cases and is now regarded as necessary for a firm diagnosis of acute rheumatic fever.

Demonstration of a high level of streptococcal antibody in the blood

ANTISTREPTOLYSIN O TEST (ASO TEST)
A level of over 200 Todd units in adults or 333 Todd units in children is found in 85% cases of rheumatic fever. A rise in titre of this antibody over several weeks is even more reliable evidence of a streptococcal infection.

RHEUMATIC FEVER PATIENTS WITH A LOW ASO TITRE
1 Very early stage of the illness. A small proportion have a low ASO titre at the first examination.
2 Late stage of the illness. Patients with chorea (onset usually 2 months or more after a streptococcal infection) have low or borderline titres.

Isolation of Group A streptococcus from the throat
Attempted culture of the streptococcus from the throat is a less satisfactory method of establishing recent streptococcal infection because:
1 Some normal individuals harbour Group A streptococci in the upper respiratory tract.
2 At the onset of rheumatic fever the streptococci may be sparse and difficult to culture from the throat.

Prognosis

1   Complete recovery—Majority of patients.
2   Permanent damage to heart valves (mitral stenosis, mitral incompetence, aortic stenosis, aortic incompetence, tricuspid stenosis and incompetence)—Small minority.
3   Congestive cardiac failure and death during the acute attack—Now rare. The severity of rheumatic fever is at present declining.
4   Recurrence of rheumatic fever—Common during childhood and early adult life.

Treatment

Bed rest
Until the patient is afebrile, gaining weight and the ESR is normal.

Salicylates
Dosage adjusted to maintain a serum salicylate level of 30 mg/100 ml (aspirin approx. 80 mg/kg body weight per day in divided doses). Joint symptoms and fever are dramatically relieved but salicylates have no effect on the incidence or severity of carditis.

Steroids
Prednisolone 10–20 mg daily is used in place of salicylates in patients with evidence of acute rheumatic carditis. Steroids reduce the severity of the acute illness but have no influence on the incidence or severity of subsequent chronic rheumatic heart disease.

Penicillin
Procaine penicillin, 600,000 units twice daily for 6 days. Elimination of the haemolytic streptococcus early in the disease reduces the severity of the acute rheumatic attack. When the diagnosis has been made late, penicillin is still indicated to eradicate any residual streptococci.

Prevention of Recurrence

Further infections with the group A streptococcus are likely to be followed by further attacks of rheumatic fever and increasing cardiac damage in susceptible patients.

Continuous prophylaxis against haemolytic streptococcal infections is advised for all patients who have suffered an attack of rheumatic fever (Penicillin V 125 mg twice daily by mouth *or* Sulphadimidine 0·5 G twice daily by mouth *or* Benzathine penicillin 1·2 mega units intramuscularly once a month).

Intramuscular benzathine penicillin is the most effective but can be painful and is reserved for those patients with serious carditis.

Prophylaxis against haemolytic streptococcal infection is continued until at least the age of 18.

CHAPTER 7
MITRAL VALVE DISEASE

MITRAL STENOSIS

Aetiology

Rheumatic

Accounts for over 99% of cases. Mitral stenosis is the most common valve lesion caused by rheumatic fever, and is four times as frequent in females as in males. The inflamed mitral valve cusps adhere at the commissures, and fibrosis and shortening of the cusps and chordae tendineae proceed for years. Fully developed cases usually appear over the age of 20.

Thirty per cent of patients with mitral stenosis have no history of rheumatic fever or chorea—the acute illness was mild and escaped notice, or has subsequently been forgotten.

Congenital

A rare lesion.

Anatomy

Rheumatic mitral stenosis

1 Commissures adherent, leaving small, oval, central orifice.
2 Cusps thickened and fibrous.
3 Chordae tendineae thickened and shortened.

Congenital mitral stenosis

The valve consists of a diaphragm with a hole in it, to which anomalous chordae tendineae are attached.

Haemodynamics (Fig. 7.1)

Rise in left atrial pressure

The narrowed mitral valve orifice obstructs blood flow through it and the left atrial pressure rises. The level to which the left atrial pressure rises is determined by the size of the mitral orifice and the blood flow per minute.

Increased passage of fluid out of the pulmonary capillaries into the lungs

The high pressure in the left atrium is transmitted to the pulmonary veins and the pulmonary capillaries, causing an increased movement of fluid into the interstitial tissues, the lymphatics and the alveoli of the lungs.

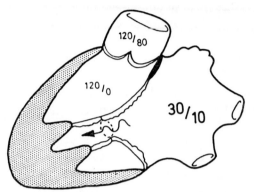

Fig. 7.1   Haemodynamics of mitral stenosis

Raised pulmonary artery pressure

The pressure in the pulmonary artery is always higher than in the pulmonary veins, and the pulmonary arterial pressure is therefore increased coincidentally with the increase in pulmonary venous pressure.

Preferential blood flow through the upper lobes

This is a reversal of the normal, when the greater part of the blood flow is through the lower zones in the upright position. Elevation of the pressure in a pulmonary vein causes constriction of the arterioles in the part of the lung drained by that vein (the mechanism for this reflex is not understood). The high left atrial pressure of mitral stenosis plus the hydrostatic pressure increases the pressure most in the lower lobe pulmonary veins. Pulmonary arterial vasoconstriction is therefore also most marked in the lower lobes and most of the pulmonary blood flow goes through the upper lobes.

Clinical Presentation of Classical Mitral Stenosis

Symptoms

A result of increased pulmonary venous pressure (p. 1) (dyspnoea on exertion; orthopnoea; paroxysmal nocturnal dyspnoea; bronchitis; haemoptysis).

Clinical examination

GENERAL
Normal facies.

BRACHIAL PULSE
Normal or rather small in amplitude.

JUGULAR VENOUS PRESSURE
Normal.

CARDIAC IMPULSES
Tapping sensation at the apex (palpable vibrations of a loud first heart sound). Diastolic thrill frequently present at apex.

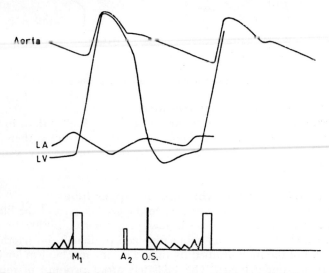

FIG. 7.2   Presystolic murmur, opening snap (O.S.) and diastolic murmur

AUSCULTATION (Fig. 7.2)

Loud first heart sound at apex
(Normally, towards the end of diastole, left ventricular filling is complete and the mitral valve cusps have drifted together so that little further movement is required from the mitral valve for complete closure. Ventricular filling has not been completed at the end of diastole when there is narrowing of the mitral valve, and the valve is still open at the commencement of ventricular systole. Considerable

movement of the valve cusps takes place in closing, the ventricle is contracting faster with the delayed valve closure, and the first sound is loud. A loud first sound is not present if the valve is rigid or extensively calcified.)

Opening snap
Heard at the apex, or between apex and left sternal edge. (Present when the fused valve cusps are mobile. The fused cusps are forced sharply down into the left ventricle by the high left atrial pressure as the left ventricular pressure falls below it, and the opening snap corresponds to the abrupt halting of the valve cone and the opening of the valve at the completion of its descent.)

Diastolic murmur
Low pitched, rumbling in character, localized to the cardiac apex, and beginning immediately after the opening snap. (Turbulent blood flow across the narrowed mitral orifice. If stenosis is severe, turbulent flow continues throughout diastole and the diastolic murmur is then of long duration.)

Presystolic murmur
Maximal at the cardiac apex—a sudden crescendo of the diastolic murmur. (Increased turbulent flow across the mitral valve during left atrial systole. The presystolic murmur is absent in atrial fibrillation.)

Electrocardiography

P MITRALE
P wave notched and 0·12 seconds or more in duration (the enlarged and hypertrophied left atrium is responsible for prolongation of the late left atrial component of the P wave).

QRS AND T COMPLEXES NORMAL
The left ventricle is small and the right ventricle is not appreciably affected when the pulmonary vascular resistance is low.

Chest X-ray
1 The left atrial appendage and the left atrium are enlarged (combination of raised left atrial pressure and a variable degree of destruction and fibrosis of the left atrial myocardium from the rheumatic process).
2 Pulmonary veins prominent, particularly in the upper zones

(high pressure in all pulmonary veins, with increased blood flow through the upper zones).

3   Lung fields show pulmonary venous congestion, often with interstitial septal lines in the costo-phrenic angles (oedema of the interlobular lung septa most marked at the lowest parts where the hydrostatic pressure is greatest).

Echocardiography
Diastolic closure rate of valve less than 70 mm/sec.

Cardiac catheterization and angiography
Not always necessary either for diagnosis or assessment of severity. The left atrial pressure is abnormally high and there is a pressure gradient between left atrium and left ventricle during diastole. The height of the left atrial pressure correlates well with the severity of the stenosis provided the cardiac output remains normal, a mean left atrial pressure over 15 mm Hg at rest indicating considerable stenosis. Angiography allows an assessment of the mobility of the valve cusps, excludes left atrial myxoma and may demonstrate left atrial thrombus, but is only used when the diagnosis is in doubt.

Important Variations in the Clinical Presentation of Mitral Stenosis

Accurate diagnosis of mitral stenosis includes an estimate of the severity of the stenosis, an evaluation of the mobility of the valve cusps, assessment of pulmonary vascular resistance and evaluation of any other valve lesions. All these factors influence management.

Severity of the stenosis

GRADES OF SEVERITY
1   Mild (valve orifice greater than 1·8 cm).   2   Moderate (valve orifice 1·5 cm).   3   Severe (valve orifice 1 cm).

ESTIMATION OF THE SEVERITY OF THE STENOSIS
The severity of the stenosis is estimated from the symptoms, clinical examination and chest X-ray (the left atrial pressures are similar in patients in any one grade and some estimate of this pressure is possible on clinical grounds).

Symptoms
The most revealing symptom is the level of activity inducing dyspnoea: Mild stenosis—dyspnoea on extraordinary effort such as running (Grade 1).

Moderate stenosis—dyspnoea walking quickly on the level, and when performing heavier household tasks—bed-making, floor-polishing, washing (Grade 2). Mild orthopnoea.

Severe stenosis—dyspnoea walking slowly (Grade 3). Severe orthopnoea, attacks of nocturnal dyspnoea. All but lightest tasks have to be abandoned.

Clinical examination

Auscultation:

1 Mild stenosis—mitral diastolic murmur occupies half diastole at normal heart rates (thereafter the pressure in the left atrium has equalized with the pressure in the left ventricle).

The opening snap is late, following A2 by more than 0·1 sec (the left atrial pressure is low and the mitral valve opens towards the end of ventricular relaxation).

2 Moderate stenosis—mitral diastolic murmur almost fills diastole. Opening snap about 0·08 sec after A2.

3 Severe stenosis—diastolic murmur extends throughout diastole, from an early opening snap (0·06 sec) up to the first heart sound (the left atrial pressure never equalizes with the left ventricular pressure during diastole).

Chest X-ray

Severe stenosis is characterized by pulmonary venous congestion and septal (Kerley's) lines. Less severe grades do not have septal lines and the lung fields are nearer normal.

Electrocardiography

If sinus rhythm is present with severe stenosis a P mitrale is the rule but it may also be seen in mild stenosis.

Cardiac catheterization

Indicated when symptoms conflict with clinical examination.

1 Mild stenosis—left atrial pressure, or wedge pressure, 5–10 mm Hg at rest, and falling to left ventricular level at the end of diastole.

2 Moderate stenosis—resting left atrial pressure over 10 mm Hg.

3 Severe stenosis—resting left atrial pressure 20 mm Hg or more, and a gradient between atrium and ventricle persisting throughout diastole.

Mobility of the valve cusps

Calcification or extensive fibrosis of the mitral valve destroys mobility.

CLINICAL FEATURES
1 Soft first heart sound (valve cusps move poorly at onset of systole, causing few audible vibrations).
2 Opening snap absent (limited valve movement).
3 Mitral calcification seen on penetrated lateral chest X-ray or on screening.

The pulmonary vascular resistance
Twenty five per cent of patients with severe mitral stenosis develop an active constriction of the pulmonary arterioles throughout the lungs, though most marked in the lower lobes. When this occurs the pulmonary arterial pressure can reach extremely high levels as the constricted pulmonary arterioles offer great resistance to blood flow. The mechanism of this reactive pulmonary hypertension is unknown, nor is it known why only 25% of patients with severe mitral stenosis respond in this way. Reactive pulmonary hypertension is not seen with mild mitral stenosis.

RAISED PULMONARY VASCULAR RESISTANCE
When the pulmonary vascular resistance is high the major obstruction to blood flow in the circulation becomes the pulmonary arterioles, and the clinical features are those of pulmonary hypertension and a low cardiac output progressing to right ventricular failure.

Symptoms
Fatigue (low cardiac output).
Ankle swelling (right ventricular failure).
Symptoms of pulmonary and systemic emboli (sluggish blood flow favours clot formation in leg veins and in left atrium).
Severe breathless attacks are now less common (low cardiac output reduces left atrial pressure).

Clinical examination
1 General. Mitral facies, cool extremities, peripheral cyanosis (low cardiac output).
2 Pulse. Small amplitude arterial pulse.
3 Jugular venous pressure. Large *a* wave (hypertrophied right ventricle requiring increased filling pressure).
4 Cardiac impulses. Parasternal heave (right ventricular hypertrophy). Palpable pulmonary second sound.
5 Auscultation.
  (i) P2 accentuated (high pulmonary artery pressure).
  (ii) Early diastolic murmur at left sternal edge (pulmonary valve regurgitation due to high pressure).

(iii) Pansystolic murmur over lower sternum increasing during inspiration (functional tricuspid regurgitation as right ventricle dilates).

(iv) Pulmonary ejection click (dilated main pulmonary artery).

(v) The apical diastolic murmur of mitral stenosis may be inaudible (blood flow across the narrowed valve is greatly reduced by the low cardiac output and makes the murmur very soft).

Electrocardiography
P pulmonale and P mitrale (combined right and left atrial enlargement).
QRS and T changes of right ventricular hypertrophy (p. 45).

Chest X-ray
Dilated main pulmonary artery (raised pulmonary arterial pressure).
Clear peripheral lung fields (smaller pulmonary arteries are constricted, particularly in the lower zones).

Pulmonary venous congestion, septal lines and left atrial enlargement are not always present (left atrial pressure may be near normal when the cardiac output is grossly reduced).

Cardiac catheterization
The mean pulmonary arterial pressure is greatly raised compared with the mean left atrial pressure (p. 83).

Other valve lesions
Mitral stenosis may be accompanied by mitral regurgitation, aortic stenosis and regurgitation and tricuspid stenosis and regurgitation.

EVIDENCE OF MITRAL REGURGITATION
Left ventricular hypertrophy (left ventricle pumps large volume of blood).
Pansystolic murmur at the apex.
Third heart sound at the apex (indicates dominant mitral regurgitation).

OTHER VALVE LESIONS
Rheumatic fever also affects the aortic valve in a considerable number of patients with mitral stenosis, and the tricuspid valve in over 5% of cases. The low cardiac output and the signs of mitral stenosis may partly obscure the evidence of lesions of these valves.

Prognosis of Mitral Stenosis

Patients with severe stenosis become completely incapacitated from dyspnoea. Furthermore incapacity and death can result from the complications of this disease:

Atrial fibrillation (develops in 40% of patients)
The patient's age and the size of the left atrium are the important factors—the older patient with a large left atrium is more likely to develop atrial fibrillation.

Systemic embolism (10% of patients)
Atrial fibrillation favours the formation of clot as does a large left atrial appendage—over 90% of major emboli in mitral stenosis occur in fibrillating patients, often within days of onset of the fibrillation. The severity of the stenosis and the size of the left atrium are less significant factors.

Recurrent embolism is common.

Reactive pulmonary hypertension (25% of patients with severe stenosis)
Death or severe disability in this group is due to:
Right ventricular failure (pressure load on right ventricle).
Pulmonary infarction and systemic embolism (low cardiac output predisposes to thrombus formation and embolism).

Acute pulmonary oedema
This is responsible for a few deaths, usually early in the course of the disease. Tachycardia during severe exertion or pregnancy is usually the precipitating factor.

Bacterial endocarditis
Uncommon in pure mitral stenosis, but frequently involves a mitral valve that has a mild regurgitant jet.

Bronchitis
Attacks of acute bronchitis and chronic bronchitis are both common in patients with mitral stenosis (congested bronchi with lowered resistance to infection).

Surgical Treatment of Mitral Stenosis

Indications for surgery
1   Moderate or severe stenosis (1·7 cm in diameter or less) causing symptoms.

2 Mitral stenosis associated with pulmonary hypertension.
3 Mitral stenosis with a high risk of systemic embolism:
 (i) The older patient in atrial fibrillation.
 (ii) When systemic embolism has already occurred.
 (iii) A large left atrial appendage. The risk of systemic embolism is trebled compared with that in the presence of a small appendage.

Mild stenosis (orifice greater than 1·8 cm in diameter) does not cause severe dyspnoea and carries only a small risk of systemic embolism except in middle aged women with atrial fibrillation. The possibility of surgical creation of mitral incompetence balances the advantages of operation in this group who are best treated with long term anticoagulation.

Surgical technique

CLOSED TRANSVENTRICULAR VALVOTOMY WITH A DILATOR (Fig. 7.3)

The classical method for uncomplicated cases. A dilator is introduced through the apex of the beating left ventricle under the control of a

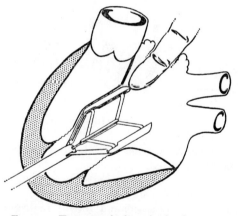

FIG. 7.3 Transventricular mitral valvotomy

finger in the left atrium and is opened in the mitral valve. Temporary bypass of the lungs during valvotomy, by taking blood from a vena cava, oxygenating it with a pump oxygenator and returning it to the femoral artery, is added if the pulmonary vascular resistance is greatly raised (Fig. 7.4).

OPEN MITRAL VALVOTOMY

May become the technique of choice when the problems of accurate

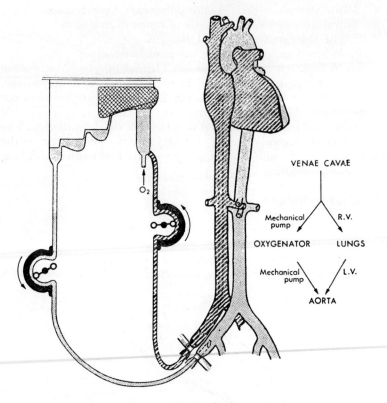

FIG. 7.4 Supportive bypass

mobilization of the cusps are mastered. Used whenever clot in the left atrium is strongly suspected.

MITRAL VALVE REPLACEMENT
Necessary when there is associated mitral regurgitation or gross calcification of the valve.

Results

MORTALITY
1 Good risk patients (mobile cusps, no associated mitral incompetence, no lesions of other valves, normal pulmonary vascular resistance)—operative mortality 3%.
2 The operative mortality of mitral valvotomy can rise as high as 30% if there is also regurgitation and calcification of the valve, a

markedly raised pulmonary vascular resistance and associated rheumatic aortic and tricuspid valve disease.

MORBIDITY

1 Significant mitral regurgitation is produced or increased in 10% of closed mitral valvotomies.

2 Systemic embolism (5%).

3 *Restenosis* of the mitral valve, due either to an inadequate initial valvotomy or to true readhesion of the commissures, affects a small number of patients in the years after mitral valvotomy.

MITRAL REGURGITATION

Aetiology and Pathology

Regurgitation of the mitral valve may be caused by disease of the mitral valve cusps, chordae tendineae, papillary muscles or valve ring.

Rheumatic
The effects of severe rheumatic fever on the mitral valve that cause mitral regurgitation are; thickening, distortion and calcification of the valve cusps allowing insufficient tissue for apposition, shortening of the chordae tendineae pulling the cusps, particularly the posterior, into the ventricle, dilatation of the valve ring, or rupture of chordae tendineae.

Subacute bacterial endocarditis
Destruction of valve tissue, perforation of a cusp or rupture of chordae tendineae lead to mitral regurgitation.

Traumatic
Blunt or penetrating injury, or an inaccurate mitral valvotomy may injure cusps, chordae or papillary muscles.

Left ventricular failure
Dilatation of the left ventricle causes dilatation of the mitral valve ring and may make the valve regurgitant. This *functional* regurgitation may disappear after treatment of the heart failure.

Myocardial infarction
Involvement of a papillary muscle in an area of infarction may cause it to rupture or function poorly and allow regurgitation.

Congenital heart disease

Congenital mitral regurgitation may be the sole lesion or accompany other congenital defects. Anatomical abnormalities include cleft valve leaflets, short aberrant chordae tendineae and papillary muscles, a dilated valve ring, or a redundant cusp ballooning into the ventricle.

Ruptured chordae tendineae

See p. 146.

Haemodynamics

To and fro movement of blood across the mitral valve
(Fig. 7.5)

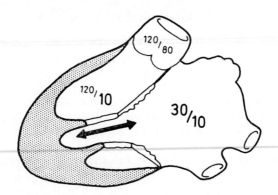

FIG. 7.5   Haemodynamics of mitral regurgitation

REGURGITANT JET THROUGHOUT SYSTOLE

Regurgitation begins with the onset of ventricular systole (M_1) and continues until the ventricular pressure falls to atrial level (i.e. after A_2) (Fig. 1.12). The forward flow into the aorta is reduced.

INCREASED FLOW DURING DIASTOLE

During diastole the blood flow from left atrium to left ventricle includes both the blood flowing into the atrium from the lungs and the blood regurgitated into the left atrium during the previous ventricular systole. The ventricle is rapidly distended until the downward movement of the apex is abruptly checked as the mitral valve cusps, chordae and papillary muscles are drawn tight. This sets up vibrations producing a third sound and, as blood continues to flow rapidly across the taut cusps, a flow murmur.

Raised left atrial and pulmonary venous pressure

There is a large v wave due to the volume of blood regurgitated into the atrium during ventricular systole. The atrial pressure at the end of diastole is similar to that in the ventricle as the valve is not obstructed. The mean left atrial pressure is therefore usually not as high as in mitral stenosis.

Left ventricular dilatation and hypertrophy

The left ventricle dilates and hypertrophies to accommodate the extra volume load.

Clinical Presentation of Rheumatic Mitral Regurgitation

Symptoms

1 Dyspnoea on exertion, orthopnoea, paroxysmal nocturnal dyspnoea, haemoptysis, bronchitis (pulmonary venous congestion).
2 Fatigue (low cardiac output).
3 Ankle oedema, hepatic pain, anorexia (secondary right ventricular failure).

Clinical examination

GENERAL
A mitral facies is less common than in mitral stenosis because the lower mean left atrial pressure causes a lower incidence of a raised pulmonary vascular resistance and consequent low cardiac output (p. 8).

PULSE
1 Rhythm—Atrial fibrillation is usual in patients with severe rheumatic mitral regurgitation.
2 Wave form—Normal or sharp (powerful left ventricular contraction).

JUGULAR VENOUS PRESSURE
Slight elevation usually—considerable elevation indicates right ventricular failure.

CARDIAC IMPULSES
Vigorous large amplitude apex beat (large overactive left ventricle).

AUSCULTATION (Fig. 7.6)
1 Pansystolic murmur blowing in character maximal at the apex and conducted to the axilla (the direction of the jet is backwards), loudest on expiration (left heart lesion).

2   Soft first sound (the cusps have floated together at the end of diastole in mitral regurgitation as the atrial and ventricular pressures have equalized by this time).
3   Third sound (rapid filling of the left ventricle in early diastole).
4   Short diastolic flow murmur following the third sound (rapid flow across the taut mitral valve cusps as the large volume from the left atrium flows into the left ventricle).

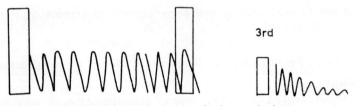

3rd

FIG. 7.6   Auscultation in mitral regurgitation

Electrocardiography
P mitrale (if in sinus rhythm). Usually atrial fibrillation.
Left ventricular hypertrophy (volume overload of left ventricle).

Chest X-ray
Enlargement of left atrium and ventricle (accommodating the increased volume). Pulmonary venous congestion and septal lines (raised left atrial pressure) are seen when the left ventricle fails.

Cardiac catheterization and angiography
Injection of contrast into the left ventricle allows approximate quantitation of mitral regurgitation into mild (jet of contrast seen entering the left atrium) and severe (marked opacification of the left atrium). Measurement of the left atrial pressure is no guide to the severity of the regurgitation because of the damping effect of a large left atrium.

Prognosis

The symptom-free period is longer than in mitral stenosis but the downhill course is rapid after the onset of left ventricular failure.
   Complications of mitral regurgitation:
1   Left ventricular failure (volume overload).
2   Systemic embolism (atrial clot) is no less common than in mitral stenosis (40%).
3   Subacute bacterial endocarditis (mild mitral regurgitation associated with sinus rhythm is the most susceptible of all lesions to endocarditis).

4   Pulmonary hypertension. Less common than in mitral stenosis (lower mean left atrial pressure).

Treatment of Mitral Regurgitation

Medical

MILD CASES
Penicillin cover for dental operations (p. 73). No other limitations.

MODERATE CASES
Digitalis and diuretics if there is any evidence of pulmonary venous congestion.

Surgery

INDICATIONS FOR SURGERY
Serious symptoms with prognosis estimated to be less than four years (the mortality and morbidity of correction of valve regurgitation does not yet warrant less stringent indications).

TECHNIQUE

Valvoplasty
If the cusps are mobile, the valve ring can be made smaller by large sutures supported by a tuck in the atrial wall. Reducing the size of the ring allows previously incompetent cusps to appose (Fig. 7.7). The plication for ruptured chordae tendineae of the posterior cusp is different (p. 148).

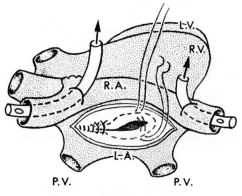

FIG. 7.7   Mitral valvoplasty

Valve replacement
Indicated for rigid and calcified cusps. A prosthesis is the best replacement today (1973) and is inserted using cardiopulmonary bypass. The exact type of prosthesis likely to give the best long term results is still being evaluated but the most consistent results are being given by cloth covered ball valves.

RESULTS

Valvoplasty
Mortality 10% in suitable cases, but subsequent recurrence of mitral regurgitation is not uncommon unless the valvoplasty is being carried out specifically for ruptured chordae of the posterior cusp (p. 148).

Prosthetic valve replacement
Immediate results good but long-term results not yet known. Complications include:
1   Operative mortality 10%.
2   Systemic embolism following thrombus formation on the prosthesis (approximately 5% of patients). Incidence markedly reduced by efficient anticoagulation after operation and the use of cloth covered frames.
3   Bacterial endocarditis.
4   Regurgitation around the valve ring.

Mitral Regurgitation due to Ruptured Chordae

Aetiology
1   Idiopathic. Occurs suddenly in middle age, often in people with systemic hypertension.
2   Bacterial endocarditis.
3   In association with mucoid degeneration of the mitral valve (redundant cusp, systolic click syndrome). The mitral valve cusps are thickened, and voluminous and the chordae long and attenuated allowing the cusps to prolapse into the atrium. May be associated with connective tissue disorders such as Ehlers-Danlos syndrome.

Incidence
20% of all patients requiring surgery for mitral regurgitation.

Clinical presentation

SYMPTOMS
Sudden onset of dyspnoea, orthopnoea. Loud heart murmur appearing in a previously normal heart.

SIGNS

If the aetiology is the redundant cusp syndrome, a mid-systolic click may have previously been heard (cause unknown).

Sinus rhythm. Pansystolic murmur and thrill at apex radiating to base of heart in rupture of posterior leaflet chordae (central part of the cusp forms a hood directing the jet anteriorly towards the root of the aorta (Fig. 7.8). Confusion with aortic stenosis may occur). Rupture of chordae to the anterior leaflet causes the murmur to radiate to the axilla as usual. Presystolic gallop rhythm (4th sound).

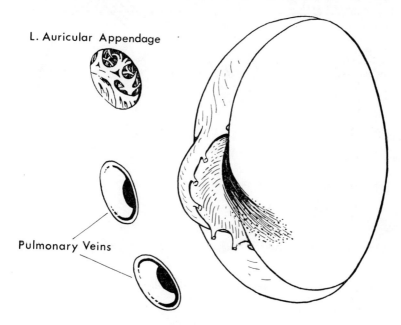

L. Auricular Appendage

Pulmonary Veins

FIG. 7.8   Rupture of chordae tendineae to posterior cusp. Regurgitant jet directed forwards

CHEST X-RAY

Small left atrium on chest X-ray.

CARDIAC CATHETERIZATION

Large v waves (over 40 mm Hg) in the left atrial pressure on cardiac catheterization.

Prognosis and treatment

Usually a progressive lesion. The regurgitation is severe and cardiac surgery is usually necessary when the diagnosis has been established.

F

Rupture of posterior leaflet chordae can be treated by plication of the leaflet so that it is supported by adjacent, still attached chordae (McGoon operation) (Fig. 7.9). Rupture of anterior leaflet chordae or rupture of chordae associated with the redundant cusp syndrome requires valve replacement.

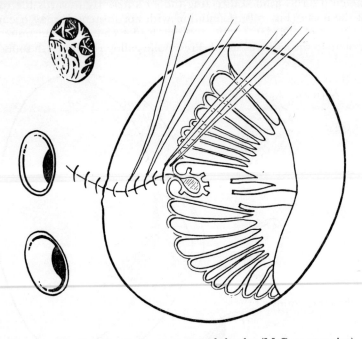

FIG. 7.9   Plication of posterior cusp ruptured chordae (McGoon operation)

CHAPTER 8
AORTIC STENOSIS AND REGURGITATION

AORTIC STENOSIS

Aortic stenosis occurs at 3 sites (Fig. 8.1): at valve level (rheumatic or congenital in origin), below the aortic valve (congenital and familial) or above the aortic valve (congenital)—rare.

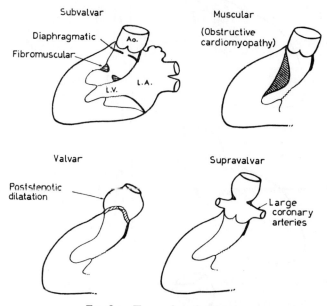

FIG. 8.1   Types of aortic stenosis

AORTIC VALVE STENOSIS

Aetiology and Pathology

Congenital

Commonly the valve is bicuspid although one of the cusps may possess a rudimentary commissure. Fusion between the two cusps produces stenosis presenting in infancy or childhood. Alternatively, stenosis may only become severe when the continued trauma to the

abnormal valve causes it to become rigid and calcified in later life
(isolated calcific aortic stenosis of adults).

Rheumatic

The rheumatic process causes fusion between the valve commissures
and thickening of the cusps. Aortic stenosis results which becomes
increasingly severe over the years as the affected valve becomes
calcified and rigid. Some aortic regurgitation is often associated with
the stenosis and the mitral valve shows evidence of rheumatic
damage.

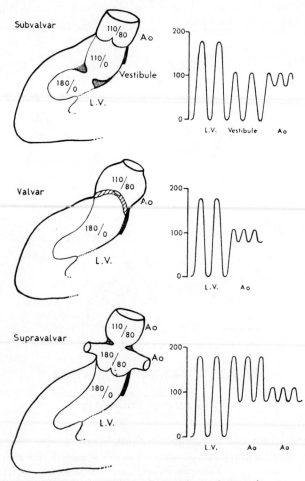

Fig. 8.2   Withdrawal traces in aortic stenosis

Haemodynamics

Systolic gradient across the valve

The pressure during left ventricular systole is higher in the left ventricle than in the aorta (Fig. 8.2).

Left ventricular hypertrophy

The increased left ventricular work necessary to eject blood through the narrowed orifice results in left ventricular hypertrophy. Left ventricular dilatation does not occur unless the ventricle fails or aortic regurgitation is present also.

Poststenotic dilatation

A localized dilatation occurs distal to the obstruction due to the lateral force on the aortic wall exerted by the turbulence of the jet of blood.

Clinical Presentation

Symptoms

ANGINA PECTORIS

Forty per cent of patients of all ages with severe aortic stenosis have angina pectoris which is indistinguishable from that due to coronary artery disease (coronary blood flow is insufficient for the needs of the hypertrophied left ventricle).

DIZZINESS AND SYNCOPE ON EFFORT

Faintness and loss of consciousness during effort indicate severe disease (the cardiac output does not rise sufficiently during exercise and cerebral blood flow is reduced). In some cases syncope is due to transient attacks of ventricular fibrillation. Sudden death during exertion is common in association with severe stenosis and may be the first indication of the disease.

DYSPNOEA

Dyspnoea on exertion indicates a rising diastolic pressure in the left ventricle transmitted to the pulmonary veins. This may progress to pulmonary oedema and eventually to congestive cardiac failure if the patient does not die earlier.

Clinical examination

GENERAL

Normal. Sometimes pale delicate complexion (*Dresden China*).

PULSE
1   Rhythm—sinus rhythm is almost invariable. Atrial fibrillation suggests associated mitral valve disease.
2   Amplitude—small.
3   Wave form—slow rising, prolonged and often with a notch on the upstroke—the *anacrotic* or *plateau* pulse.

BLOOD PRESSURE
Systolic pressure slightly reduced. Pulse pressure small.

JUGULAR VENOUS PRESSURE
Normal.

CARDIAC IMPULSES
Marked left ventricular hypertrophy. Systolic thrill felt over the aortic area and carotid arteries.

AUSCULTATION (Fig. 8.3)
1   Loud ejection murmur heard at aortic area, over carotid arteries, and often well heard at the apex (turbulence of blood flowing through the stenotic valve at a high velocity).
2   Ejection click (valve dome arrested sharply in its fully open position). If the ejection click is absent, it suggests that either the valve is rigid and calcified or the stenosis is not at valve level.
3   Second sound (Fig. 8.3).

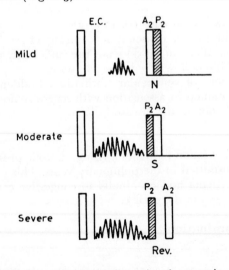

FIG. 8.3   Auscultation in aortic valve stenosis

(i) Mild stenosis. Narrowly split during inspiration and single on expiration (only slight prolongation of left ventricular ejection time).

(ii) Moderate stenosis. Single second sound (left ventricular systole is prolonged so that on expiration the aortic second sound (A_2) falls immediately after the pulmonary (P_2), and the sounds are heard as one. On inspiration P_2 is delayed and moves across A_2 but the gap is small between them so that the sound remains single to the ear). If the valve is calcified, the second sound is single because A_2 is inaudible and only P_2 is heard.

(iii) Severe stenosis. Reversed second sound (left ventricular systole is considerably prolonged and on expiration A_2 falls well after P_2 making the sound split. On inspiration the normal delay of P_2 makes it fall close to A_2 and the second sound becomes single—i.e. the sound behaves in a reversed manner to the normal).

Electrocardiography
Left ventricular hypertrophy and strain (p. 44), the degree correlating reasonably well with the severity of the stenosis except in children, in whom the E.C.G. may be normal in the presence of severe aortic stenosis.

Chest X-ray
1 The transverse diameter of the heart is not increased unless left ventricular failure has occurred or there is associated aortic regurgitation (hypertrophy of the left ventricle without dilatation is not visible on the chest X-ray).
2 Poststenotic dilatation of the ascending aorta.
3 Calcification in a stenosed aortic valve is invariable in patients over the age of forty, except occasionally when the aetiology is rheumatic. The absence of calcification in patients of this age group is against the diagnosis of valve stenosis.

Cardiac catheterization and angiography
Used to determine accurately the site and severity of the stenosis and the presence of associated mitral valve and coronary arterial disease. A catheter is placed in the left ventricle for pressure measurements and the injection of radio-opaque contrast fluid. The catheter is passed either trans-septally or retrograde across the aortic valve from the femoral or brachial artery (difficult when the stenosis is severe).

SEVERITY
Assessed by simultaneous pressure measurements in left ventricle and aorta together with a measurement of the cardiac output (Fig. 8.2).

The more severe the stenosis, the greater the systolic pressure difference between the left ventricle and the aorta. The area of the aortic valve orifice can be calculated from the formula:

$$\text{Aortic orifice area} = 44\cdot5 \sqrt{\frac{\text{Mean systolic flow in ml/sec}}{\text{mean systolic pressure gradient between L.V. and aorta}}}$$

SITE OF STENOSIS

Angiocardiography shows the exact anatomy of the stenosis. In addition, if the retrograde method of catheterization is used, a single change of pressure is seen as the catheter is withdrawn from left ventricle to aorta (Fig. 8.2).

PRESENCE OF MITRAL VALVE DISEASE

Mitral stenosis
Trans-septal catheterization shows a pressure gradient across the mitral valve during ventricular diastole.

Mitral regurgitation
The regurgitation of radio-opaque contrast into the left atrium following selective left ventricular angiography is the most reliable method for the detection of mitral regurgitation.

CORONARY ARTERY DISEASE
Frequently coexists in elderly patients. Coronary arteriography is used routinely in some centres prior to aortic valve surgery because severe coronary arterial disease will influence management.

Prognosis and Complications

Severe aortic stenosis renders the patient liable to sudden death and occasionally this is the first symptom. Symptoms of angina pectoris or syncope due to aortic stenosis are particularly ominous, the average life expectancy from their onset being 3–4 years.

Causes of death: ventricular fibrillation, left ventricular failure, bacterial endocarditis.

Treatment

Non-calcified congenital aortic stenosis

INDICATIONS FOR SURGERY
Severe stenosis is characterized by symptoms of angina and syncope,

or a systolic gradient of more than 50 mm Hg across the aortic valve when the cardiac output is normal.

TECHNIQUE
Open valvotomy using cardiopulmonary bypass and coronary artery perfusion (Fig. 8.4). Care is taken to divide the commissures accurately to avoid regurgitation.

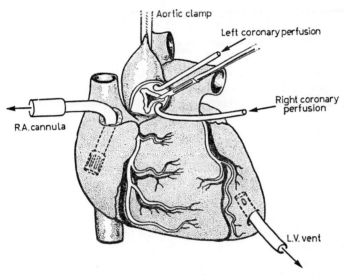

FIG. 8.4   Aortic valvotomy

RESULTS
Immediate results in terms of mortality (2%) and relief of gradient are good, but it is difficult to believe that these deformed, thickened valves will not eventually calcify and restenose.

Calcific aortic stenosis

INDICATIONS
As for non-calcific aortic stenosis.

TECHNIQUE
Replacement of the aortic valve using cardiopulmonary bypass with coronary artery perfusion. The replacement valves at present available (1973) are homografts and pulmonary valve autografts (Fig. 8.8) and prosthetic ball valve and disc prostheses (Starr, Beall, Bjork-Shiley etc.) (Fig. 8.9).

RESULTS

The operative mortality is approximately 10%. Late complications account for a further 10% mortality and include bacterial endocarditis, embolism from thrombosis on the valve, haemolytic anaemia, calcification and cusp rupture of homografts and mechanical deterioration of prostheses.

SUPRAVALVAR AORTIC STENOSIS

Anatomy

Stenosis above the aortic valve may be a narrow ring (Fig. 8.1), a longer hourglass deformity or a hypoplastic ascending aorta. Supravalvar stenosis is commonly associated with mental retardation and a peculiar facies which is also found in infantile hypercalcaemia. The coronary arteries lie below the obstruction and are very large unless they are involved in the hypoplastic process.

Clinical Presentation

The symptoms and signs are the same as in aortic valve stenosis with the following exceptions:

1   Characteristic facies in 50% (broad forehead, wide set eyes and pointed chin).

2   Left brachial pulse smaller than right (origin of left subclavian artery often narrowed).

3   No ejection click.

4   No poststenotic dilatation of the ascending aorta and no calcification of the aortic valve on the chest X-ray.

5   Withdrawal of a catheter across the stenosis shows the systolic gradient to occur in the aorta (Fig. 8.2).

6   Angiography delineates the type of supravalvar stenosis.

Treatment

Indications

Severe narrowing of the aorta.

Technique

1   Narrow ring or hourglass deformity—longitudinal incision and patch to enlarge lumen (Fig. 8.5).

2   Hypoplastic ascending aorta—replace ascending aorta with graft.

SUBVALVAR AORTIC STENOSIS
Anatomy

Stenosis in the vestibule of the left ventricle below the aortic valve is of three types:

1 Subaortic diaphragm (Fig. 8.1). A thin membrane situated just below the valve with a central hole.

2 Fibromuscular (Fig. 8.1). A narrow fibromuscular ring extending from the aortic leaflet of the mitral valve to the ventricular septum 1–2 cm below the aortic valve.

3 Muscular (hypertrophic obstructive cardiomyopathy) (Fig. 8.1). Gross and often asymmetrical hypertrophy of the ventricular septum which obstructs the ventricular outflow. It tends to be familial in incidence and its cause is unknown.

Clinical Presentation of Subaortic Diaphragmatic and Fibromuscular Stenosis

The symptoms are identical with those of aortic valve stenosis. The signs are similar but the following features suggest that the stenosis is not at valve level:

1 No ejection click.

2 No poststenotic dilatation of the ascending aorta and no calcification of the aortic valve on the chest X-ray.

3 A soft early diastolic murmur is common in both valvar and subvalvar stenosis and is of little help in the diagnosis.

4 The systolic gradient occurs in the ventricle (Fig. 8.2).

5 Left ventricular angiography shows the anatomy of the stenosis clearly.

Clinical Presentation of Hypertrophic Obstructive Cardiomyopathy

Symptoms
Appear at any age. Angina pectoris, syncope on exertion, congestive heart failure, and sudden death. There is a history of cardiomyopathy and sudden death in near relatives in about 50% of cases.

Clinical examination
The arterial pulse is abnormally fast rising (the obstruction to left ventricular outflow only begins towards the end of systole).

There is marked left ventricular hypertrophy on palpation with a double thrust at the apex.

The systolic ejection murmur is usually late in systole, best heard at the left sternal edge and not well conducted to the carotid arteries. An aortic diastolic murmur is rare.

Cardiac catheterization and angiocardiography

The pressure gradient between the left ventricle and aorta can be increased by isoprenaline, glyceryl trinitrate and digitalis, and reduced by a β adrenergic blocking drug and phenylephrine. Angiography shows the deformed, hypertrophied left ventricle with a minute cavity at the end of systole.

Treatment of Subaortic Stenosis

Subaortic diaphragmatic and fibromuscular types

INDICATIONS FOR SURGERY
Severe obstruction (as for valvar stenosis).

TECHNIQUE (Fig. 8.5)
Excision of obstruction from above through the aortic valve using cardiopulmonary bypass and avoiding damage to the mitral valve and the conduction bundle in the ventricular septum.

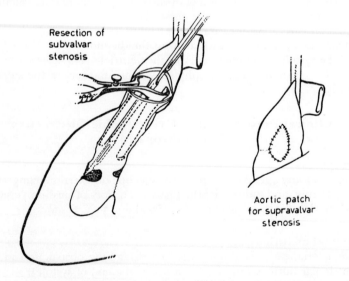

Resection of
subvalvar
stenosis

Aortic patch
for supravalvar
stenosis

FIG. 8.5   Correction of subvalvar and supravalvar aortic stenosis

RESULTS
Initially good (mortality 2%) but aortic valve regurgitation may develop later if the support of the aortic valve cusps has been weakened by removing the subvalvar obstruction.

Hypertrophic obstructive cardiomyopathy
Beta adrenergic blocking agents (propranolol etc.) may relieve the symptoms.

SURGERY

Indications
Symptoms and signs of severe obstruction unresponsive to a prolonged trial of β blocking agent.

Technique
Deep longitudinal incision through outflow tract muscle and removal of hypertrophied muscle piecemeal through an aortic incision using cardiopulmonary bypass and coronary artery perfusion.

Results
Mortality 10–25%. The symptoms and gradient are usually relieved.

AORTIC REGURGITATION

Aetiology
Rheumatic fever, bacterial endocarditis, syphilis, aneurysm of the ascending aorta, ankylosing spondylitis, ruptured aortic cusp, myxomatous degeneration of aortic valve cusps, hypertensive dilatation of the aortic root.

Rheumatic fever
Rheumatic fever may involve the aortic valve cusps leaving them shrunken, distorted and fibrotic, and usually also produces some fusion in the region of the commissures.

Bacterial endocarditis
Any lesion of the aortic valve (congenital, rheumatic, syphilitic) can be the site for bacterial invasion. A previously healthy aortic valve may be involved by spread of bacterial endocarditis from an infected mitral valve, or from an infected ventricular septal defect.

Bacterial endocarditis produces or intensifies aortic regurgitation by destroying valve tissue—perforations of one or more cusps are characteristic of bacterial endocarditis.

Syphilis
Spirochaetal infection of the aorta, the aortic valve ring and the coronary artery ostia become apparent in the tertiary stage of the disease. Severe and progressive aortic regurgitation ensues as the aortic ring dilates. Since the syphilitic process does not produce fusion of the valve cusps there is no aortic stenosis.

Congenital weakness of the aortic media and dissecting aneurysm of the aorta
A weakness of the aortic media occurs both as an isolated finding, and as part of a generalized abnormality of connective tissue in Marfan's syndrome. Progressive aneurysmal dilatation of the aorta may result in stretching of valve cusps and aortic regurgitation.

Alternatively a dissecting aneurysm may form in cystic medionecrosis in the aortic media, and when the dissection reaches the region of the aortic valve cusps the attachment of the valve to the aortic wall is loosened and it then prolapses into the ventricle causing aortic regurgitation.

Ruptured aortic cusp
Trauma to the chest wall with rupture of a valve cusp is an unusual cause of aortic valve regurgitation.

Ankylosing spondylitis and Reiter's disease
The cardiovascular system is involved in a small proportion of patients, the clinical manifestations including heart block and aortic regurgitation from dilatation of the aortic ring.

Stretch lesions of valves
Occurs in Marfan syndrome and aortic dilatation. The aortic and mitral leaflets stretch and overshoot on closing with consequent aortic or mitral regurgitation.

Haemodynamics (Fig. 8.6)

Regurgitant jet in diastole
During diastole the left ventricle is filled by blood leaking through the aortic valve in addition to that received from the left atrium. The left ventricle dilates and hypertrophies to accommodate the increased diastolic volume.

Increased stroke volume in systole

With each contraction the left ventricle ejects its increased volume of blood, but only a proportion is effective forward flow to the periphery, the remainder returning to the ventricle during diastole. The duration of ventricular systole is normal, and the increased stroke volume is ejected more rapidly, causing a fast rate of rise of arterial pressure and an aortic systolic flow murmur.

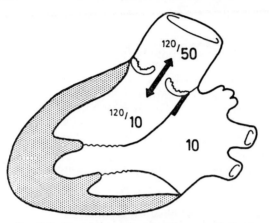

FIG. 8.6 Haemodynamics of aortic regurgitation

Clinical Presentation

Symptoms

Free aortic regurgitation can be symptomless provided that it has been of gradual onset. Acute left ventricular failure occurs at the onset of any sudden severe regurgitation since the left ventricle has had no time to adapt to the increased work load.

When aortic regurgitation produces symptoms they indicate left ventricular failure—dyspnoea, orthopnoea, paroxysmal nocturnal dyspnoea, pulmonary oedema.

Angina pectoris is uncommon, except in syphilitic regurgitation where there is interference with coronary flow due to narrowing of the coronary ostia.

Clinical examination

PULSE

1 Sinus rhythm (atrial fibrillation suggests that rheumatic involvement of the mitral valve is also present).

2 Large amplitude (high systolic, low diastolic blood pressures).

3   Water hammer character (rapid rise of pressure wave to a poorly sustained peak, with rapid fall, caused by the ejection of a large volume into a relatively empty arterial tree).
4   Abrupt distension and collapse of carotid arteries (Corrigan's sign).
5   Capillary pulsation in nail beds, and pulsation of retinal arterioles in the optic fundi (arterial pulsation transmitted to the arterioles and capillaries).

BLOOD PRESSURE
High systolic, low diastolic pressure.

JUGULAR VENOUS PRESSURE
Normal until the onset of cardiac failure.

CARDIAC IMPULSES
The apex beat is outside the mid clavicular line, abrupt, and of large amplitude in its movement (characteristic of a hypertrophied and dilated left ventricle ejecting a large volume at each stroke).

AUSCULTATION (Fig. 8.7)
1   Early diastolic murmur of regurgitation through the aortic valve—blowing, high pitched, beginning immediately after the second heart sound, loudest at the 3rd and 4th left intercostal spaces close to the sternum, but usually also heard in the aortic area and at the cardiac apex.

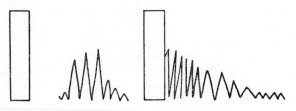

FIG. 8.7   Auscultation in aortic regurgitation

2   Systolic ejection murmur from the large volume flow into the aorta during systole. Loudest in the aortic area and propagated into the carotid arteries, this murmur is usually present even when the lesion is pure regurgitation.
3   Low rumbling presystolic or middiastolic murmur at the apex (Austin Flint murmur). The regurgitant aortic jet pushes the anterior leaflet of the mitral valve backwards, causing vibration of that valve during the inflow of atrial blood in diastole.

Electrocardiogram
Left ventricular hypertrophy.

Chest X-ray
Increased transverse diameter of the heart (dilated left ventricle).
Dilatation of ascending aorta, aortic knuckle and descending thoracic
aorta (increased blood flow to and fro between left ventricle and
aorta).

Ultrasound
Very useful for distinguishing an Austin Flint murmur from organic
mitral stenosis. In severe regurgitation the mitral valve echo shows
early closure.

Variation in Presentation with Different Aetiology

Rheumatic
A history of rheumatic fever, or the presence of atrial fibrillation and
mitral valve disease in addition to the signs of aortic regurgitation,
suggests a rheumatic aetiology.

Bacterial endocarditis
History of recent dental extraction in 50%, with the sudden onset of
aortic regurgitation accompanied by symptoms and signs of a
generalized systemic illness and a positive blood culture. Aortic
diastolic murmur often inaudible, the clues to the diagnosis being
sudden onset of failure, a loud gallop rhythm and early closure of the
mitral valve seen on ultrasound examination.

Syphilitic
Signs of syphilis in other systems, calcification of the ascending aorta
in the chest X-ray and a positive Wasserman reaction in the blood.

Dissecting aneurysm
Onset accompanied by tearing pain in chest and back, with absence
of some peripheral arterial pulses.

Aneurysm of ascending aorta due to genetic weakness
Often features of Marfan's syndrome—tall, long thin fingers,
hypermobile joints, arched palate, deformed teeth, spinal deformi-
ties, dislocation of lens of eye, abnormal metacarpal index.

Ankylosing spondylitis
Typical radiological changes in sacro-iliac joints.

Prognosis

Moderate degrees of aortic regurgitation are tolerated for many years without symptoms, and avoidance of sustained strenuous physical exertion will allow many to live a nearly normal life span.

Severe degrees of aortic regurgitation sooner or later result in intractable left ventricular failure, with an average interval of less than 1 year from the onset of failure to death.

Sudden onset as in bacterial endocarditis may require early valve replacement because of severe heart failure.

Treatment

Medical

1 Left ventricular failure is treated along the usual lines with rest, digoxin, and diuretics.

2 Bacterial endocarditis. Ideally the infection should have been eradicated for three months before undertaking surgery on the affected valve in order to allow the oedematous tissues to become fibrous and so hold sutures better. Urgent surgery because of severe heart failure is often necessary much sooner.

3 Syphilitic aortic disease is treated with penicillin.

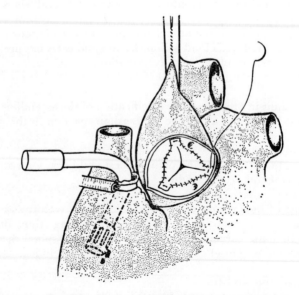

FIG. 8.8 Aortic valve replacement—homograft

Surgery

INDICATIONS FOR AORTIC VALVE REPLACEMENT
1 Serious progressive increase in heart size or deterioration of the electrocardiogram.
2 Evidence of left ventricular failure e.g. an attack of pulmonary oedema.
3 Angina pectoris.

TECHNIQUE
Using cardiopulmonary bypass the ascending aorta is occluded and opened, with perfusion of the coronary arteries to preserve the myocardium. The aortic valve is excised and replaced with either a prosthesis (Fig. 8.9) or homograft valve (Fig. 8.8).

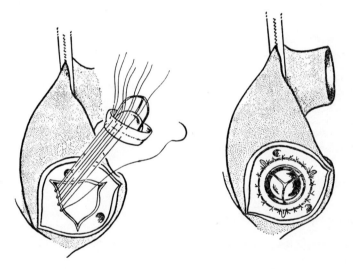

FIG. 8.9   Aortic valve replacement—Starr ball valve

RESULTS
1 Operative mortality around 10%.
2 Late mortality 10% from—bacterial endocarditis; systemic embolism and haemolytic anaemia (particularly from prosthetic valves); recurrence of regurgitation (particularly with aortic homografts).
3 Long-term results. Information on long-term function suggests

that after five years homograft valves become rigid and crack. Current developments in prosthetic valves include the use of totally cloth covered frames and metal balls and pyrolite carbon discs to reduce the risks of embolism and ball variance.

CHAPTER 9
PULMONARY STENOSIS AND REGURGITATION

PULMONARY VALVE STENOSIS

Aetiology

Congenital

Pulmonary valve stenosis is almost always congenital in origin and accounts for about 10% of all congenital heart disease. The valve is either bicuspid or tricuspid and thickened, with the cusps fused at their commissures.

Rheumatic

Pulmonary valve involvement is rare.

Carcinoid syndrome

Carcinoid tumours of the small bowel with secondary tumours in the liver secrete serotonin which is possibly the cause of the thickening, fibrosis and narrowing of the valves in the right side of the heart seen in this rare condition.

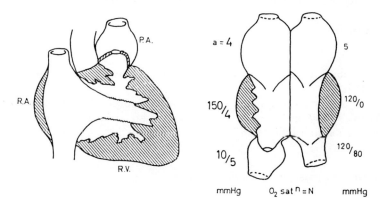

Fig. 9.1   Anatomy and haemodynamics of pulmonary valve stenosis

Haemodynamics (Fig. 9.1)

Right ventricular hypertrophy

The right ventricular pressure is raised during systole in order to overcome the obstruction to outflow, and the ventricle hypertrophies. Right atrial hypertrophy occurs to overcome the increased resistance to filling of the hypertrophied right ventricle.

Poststenotic dilatation of the pulmonary artery

The segment of the pulmonary artery immediately above the stenosed valve is dilated because of the vibration set up in the artery by the turbulence of the jet of blood. The pulmonary artery pressure is low.

Cardiac output reduced

The cardiac output is reduced by the obstruction to the circulation and this is the main haemodynamic disturbance in severe cases.

Clinical Presentation

Usually presents as an asymptomatic patient with a loud pulmonary ejection murmur and large pulmonary artery on chest X-ray.

Symptoms

Symptoms are rarely prominent in pulmonary stenosis unless the stenosis is severe, when fatigue (low cardiac output), dyspnoea (reflex response to the low cardiac output), angina (gross right ventricular hypertrophy may exceed the coronary oxygen-carrying capacity) and syncope (probably due to arrhythmias) occur.

Clinical examination

GENERAL
1 Rounding of the facial contours is common in pulmonary stenosis.
2 Cyanosis is peripheral (if the cardiac output is very low), *or* central (only in severe cases if there is an atrial communication through which blood can be shunted into the left atrium).

PULSE
Normal or small (low cardiac output).

JUGULAR VENOUS PRESSURE
Giant *a* wave (right atrial hypertrophy).

CARDIAC IMPULSES
Marked right ventricular hypertrophy. Thrill over pulmonary area.

AUSCULTATION (Fig. 9.2)

Mild stenosis (right ventricular systolic pressure 30–50 mm Hg)
Ejection click (valve dome opening sharply into dilated artery).
Relatively short ejection murmur (not much obstruction). Normal
second sound (right ventricular systole not prolonged).

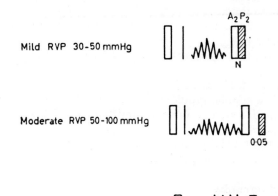

FIG. 9.2   Auscultation in pulmonary valve stenosis

Moderate stenosis (R.V. pressure 50–100 mm Hg)
Ejection click during expiration only (atrial contraction transmitted
through the right ventricle raises the pulmonary valve into the open
position before systole begins. This effect occurs during inspiration
when the flow through the right ventricle is greatest). Murmur longer
(obstruction more severe). P_2 delayed (right ventricular systole prolonged by obstruction to emptying) and soft (pulmonary artery
pressure reduced).

Severe stenosis (R.V. pressure over 150 mm Hg)
Atrial sound (right atrial hypertrophy). Ejection click disappears
(atrial contraction raises the pulmonary valve into the open position
before ventricular systole begins). Murmur very long running
through A_2, with P_2 inaudible or very late and soft (right ventricular
systole prolonged and pulmonary artery pressure low).

Electrocardiography
1   P pulmonale (tall sharp P wave over 2·5 mm in height indicating

augmentation of the initial component of the P wave due to right atrial hypertrophy).

2 Right ventricular hypertrophy (p. 45).

Chest X-ray

1 Prominent pulmonary artery (poststenotic dilatation).

2 The ventricular mass is normal (the right ventricle is hypertrophied, not dilated).

3 The lung fields tend to be abnormally clear (decreased pulmonary blood flow).

4 Enlargement of right atrium (raised right atrial pressure).

Cardiac catheterization (Fig. 9.1)

1 There is a systolic gradient across the pulmonary valve (raised right ventricular systolic pressure and lowered pulmonary arterial systolic pressure).

2 Raised right atrial pressure, particularly the *a* wave.

3 Reduced cardiac output in severe cases.

Angiocardiography

Contrast is injected into the right ventricle. The narrowed dome-shaped pulmonary valve is seen with a jet of contrast flowing through it into a dilated main pulmonary artery. The right ventricular wall is thick and may narrow the infundibulum below the valve.

Prognosis

Severe cases

Average age of death 25 years (right ventricular failure, bacterial endocarditis, cardiac arrhythmias).

Moderate cases

Bacterial endocarditis is the main danger, but persistent right ventricular hypertrophy proceeds to fibrosis and irreversible damage if the pressure is not reduced before the age of 20.

Treatment

Surgical relief of the stenosis is the only effective treatment.

Indications for surgery

1 Increasing or already marked right ventricular hypertrophy on the electrocardiogram.

2   A right ventricular systolic pressure above 70 mm Hg at rest or 100 mm Hg on effort.

Symptoms are no guide to the severity of pulmonary valve stenosis.

Technique of pulmonary valvotomy

1   Open pulmonary valvotomy through the pulmonary artery using cardiopulmonary bypass (Fig. 9.3).

(i) Closure of any atrial communication, whatever the size, as right to left shunts may otherwise persist.

(ii) Excision of the hypertrophied infundibulum if it is severe.

2   Closed pulmonary valvotomy (Brock operation) is sometimes performed for a patient in severe heart failure (Fig. 9.3), but this operation is usually confined to Fallot's Tetralogy.

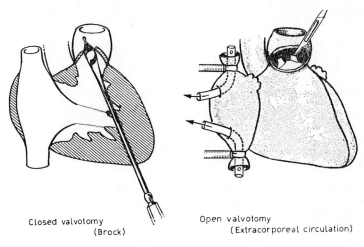

Closed valvotomy
(Brock)

Open valvotomy
(Extracorporeal circulation)

FIG. 9.3   Pulmonary valvotomy

Results

MORTALITY
2–5%.

INVOLUTION OF RIGHT VENTRICULAR HYPERTROPHY
Almost complete after two years if the stenosis is adequately relieved and the operation has been performed before the age of 20.

INFUNDIBULAR PULMONARY STENOSIS

Embryology

The ridge between bulbus (infundibulum) and primitive ventricle (body of right ventricle) persists, instead of being absorbed, and narrows the lumen (Fig. 9.4). A small ventricular septal defect is a common associated anomaly.

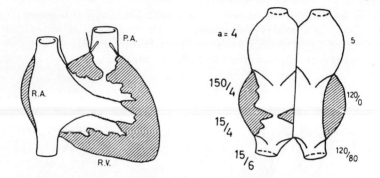

Fig. 9.4   Anatomy and haemodynamics in infundibular stenosis

Clinical Presentation

The symptoms and signs of an obstructed right ventricle are the same as in pulmonary valve stenosis, but the signs peculiar to the valve stenosis itself are absent i.e.

1   No ejection click on auscultation (Fig. 9.5).

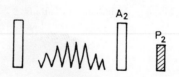

Fig. 9.5   Auscultation in infundibular stenosis

2   No poststenotic dilatation of the pulmonary artery on the chest X-ray.

3   The gradient is at infundibular level on cardiac catheterization (Fig. 9.4), and the obstruction is visualized in the ventricle by angiocardiography.

Treatment

Indications for surgery
As for pulmonary valve stenosis.

Technique of infundibular resection
With cardiopulmonary bypass the infundibulum is resected through a transverse ventriculotomy (Fig. 9.6) and any small V.S.D. closed.

Mortality
10%.

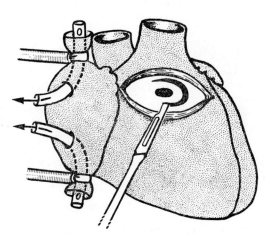

Fig. 9.6   Infundibular resection

FALLOT'S TETRALOGY

Definition

Fallot's Tetralogy is best defined as a cyanosed patient with a large ventricular septal defect and severe pulmonary stenosis (Fig. 9.7), although the spectrum varies from an acyanotic patient with a left to right shunt to a deeply cyanosed patient with pulmonary atresia.

Embryology

Fallot's Tetralogy is the result of arrest of the normal absorption of the bulbus cordis (infundibulum) into the primitive right ventricle (body of ventricle), (see p. 191):

1   The ridge between bulbus and ventricle persists (infundibular stenosis).

2   The membranous septum fails to close (ventricular septal defect).

3   There is incomplete torsion of the great arteries (overriding aorta).

4   The right ventricle hypertrophies to overcome the obstruction.

Haemodynamics

The important features of Fallot's Tetralogy are the severe pulmonary stenosis and the large ventricular septal defect (Fig. 9.7).

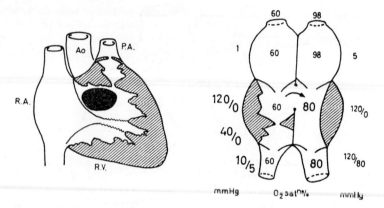

Fig. 9.7   Anatomy and haemodynamics of Fallot's Tetralogy

Severe pulmonary stenosis
The pulmonary stenosis may be at the level of the infundibulum, pulmonary valve, pulmonary artery or any combination of the three, and the resistance to blood flow of the stenosed orifice is greater than the systemic resistance.

Large ventricular septal defect
The ventricular septal defect is characteristically so large that the situation is functionally a common ventricle and both ventricular pressures are identical under all circumstances.

Right to left shunt
Blood takes the course of least resistance and venous blood passes across the defect into the systemic circulation causing central cyanosis. Alteration of the relative resistances alters the magnitude of the shunt. Increasing the infundibular tone by emotional crises, or

lowering the systemic resistance by exercise, increases the right to left shunt and the cyanosis. Relaxing infundibular tone with morphine, or raising the systemic resistance by vasopressor drugs and squatting, decreases the shunt and the cyanosis.

Low pulmonary artery pressure

The pulmonary blood flow is reduced, so that the pulmonary arteries are small and bronchial arterial collateral vessels are stimulated to join them.

Clinical Presentation

Presents as a cyanosed child with a history of squatting and syncopal attacks, moderate right ventricular hypertrophy, and a pulmonary bay and ischaemic lung fields on the chest X-ray.

Symptoms

CYANOSIS
Cyanosis is present at birth in severe cases, although in less severe cases the cyanosis becomes obvious only after a few months.

CYANOTIC ATTACKS
Sudden syncope, often during an emotional upset. The child is unconscious, deeply cyanosed or pallid with a very low arterial oxygen saturation (e.g. 20%), a normal blood pressure and an absent pulmonary ejection murmur (spasm of the infundibulum, provoked in some patients by neurogenic stimuli, profoundly reduces blood flow into the pulmonary artery. The lack of oxygenation of the blood results in syncope and even death from cerebral anoxia unless pulmonary flow is restored).

SQUATTING
Sitting on the heels after exercise with the knees bent up to the chest, appearing about the age the child begins to walk but rarely persisting into adult life (the systemic resistance is lowered on exercise, increasing the right to left shunt and the cyanosis. Squatting compresses the abdominal aorta and femoral arteries and raises the systemic resistance, decreasing the right to left shunt across the ventricular septal defect).

DYSPNOEA ON EXERTION
Due to the effect of the low arterial oxygen tension on the respiratory centre, directly and via chemoreceptors in the aortic arch and carotid body.

Clinical examination

GENERAL
Features of a right to left shunt are central cyanosis, clubbing of the fingers and polycythaemia.

PULSE AND BLOOD PRESSURE
Normal.

JUGULAR VENOUS PRESSURE
Normal or slightly raised (the right ventricle is only moderately hypertrophied and does not require a high filling pressure).

CARDIAC IMPULSES
Right ventricular hypertrophy is only moderate (the presence of a large V.S.D. ensures that the right ventricular pressure is always equal to the left ventricular pressure, unlike pure pulmonary stenosis where high right ventricular pressures are common, particularly during exercise).

AUSCULTATION (Fig. 9.8)
1   Short pulmonary ejection murmur (turbulent flow across the narrowed pulmonary infundibulum or valve).
2   Single second sound (only aortic closure is heard. P₂ is very late and inaudible because of the low pulmonary artery pressure).

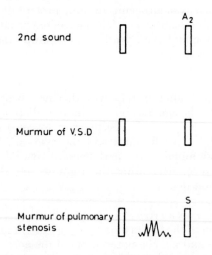

FIG. 9.8   Auscultation in Fallot's Tetralogy

3   No murmur is produced by the ventricular septal defect (which is so large that there is no turbulence as blood passes across it from right to left).

Electrocardiography
Right axis deviation and moderate right ventricular hypertrophy (right ventricular pressure never exceeds systemic).

Chest X-ray
1   Normal sized heart.
2   Absence of normal bulge of pulmonary artery (main pulmonary artery small because of the diminished blood flow through it).
3   Lung fields abnormally clear (diminished blood flow through lungs).
4   Aortic arch right sided in 25% of cases.

Cardiac catheterization (Fig. 9.7)
1   The right and left ventricular pressures are the same at all times, including exercise (large ventricular septal defect).
2   A systolic gradient is found at the level of the infundibulum or pulmonary valve and the pulmonary artery pressure is very low.
3   Left atrial blood is fully saturated but the oxygen saturation of the aortic blood is decreased by the right to left shunt.

Angiocardiography
Contrast is injected into the right ventricle and demonstrates the anatomy of the obstruction in the infundibulum or pulmonary valve. Some contrast also passes from the right ventricle through the ventricular septal defect into the aorta and outlines the defect.

Prognosis

Patients rarely survive to middle age and usually die in childhood in a cyanotic attack or from cerebral abscess.

Other complications are paradoxical embolism (venous thrombus entering the systemic circulation through the septal defect), cerebral thrombosis (polycythaemia increases the viscosity of the blood), and, less commonly, bacterial endocarditis.

Treatment

Indications for surgery
All cases of Fallot's Tetralogy should ideally be operated upon because of the above prognosis.

Surgical technique

SEVERELY ILL INFANT

Waterston anastomosis (ascending aorta/pulmonary artery shunt (Fig. 9.9)). A small anastomosis is made between ascending aorta and right pulmonary artery. Total correction is being carried out increasingly often in infancy with limited bypass and profound hypothermia.

OLDER CHILD WITH SEVERE PULMONARY STENOSIS

Severe cyanosis, packed cell volume more than 60%, haemoglobin more than 20G%, pulmonary artery less than half the size of the aorta:

1   Blalock operation (subclavian/pulmonary artery anastomosis). The pulmonary blood flow is increased by anastomosing the right or left subclavian artery to the P.A. (Fig. 9.9). The increased pulmonary blood flow enlarges the pulmonary arteries but may cause the right ventricular outflow tract to become smaller or even be obliterated altogether. For this reason a Brock operation has been recommended by some surgeons in this age group.

2   Brock operation (closed pulmonary valvotomy through the right ventricle (Fig. 9.3) with excision of the infundibular stenosis with a special punch (Fig. 9.9)). The Brock operation relieves the cyanosis and causes dilatation of the right ventricular outflow tract, facilitat-

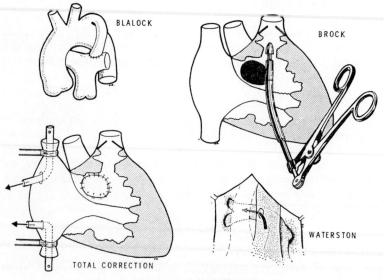

BLALOCK

BROCK

TOTAL CORRECTION

WATERSTON

FIG. 9.9   Operations for Fallot's Tetralogy

ing subsequent total correction. Total correction is often not recommended as the initial step because of the high mortality in this severe group, but is carried out within two years of the valvotomy.

OLDER CHILD WITH MODERATE PULMONARY STENOSIS
Total correction. Open pulmonary valvotomy and infundibular resection on cardiopulmonary bypass, patching the ventricular septal defect (Fig. 9.9).

Mortality
1 Waterston-Cooley anastomosis for severely cyanosed infant—40% under 6 months of age, 10% after.
2 Blalock and Brock operation—10%.
3 Total correction for moderate stenosis—10%.

Variants of Fallot's Tetralogy

Acyanotic Fallot's Tetralogy

ANATOMY
Anatomically Fallot's Tetralogy (pulmonary stenosis and large ventricular septal defect resulting functionally in a common ventricle situation) but with the pulmonary stenosis mild enough to allow a small left to right shunt at rest.

CLINICAL PRESENTATION
The child is cyanosed only on effort, and does not squat nor have syncopal attacks. Clinical examination is as in cyanotic Fallot's Tetralogy except for:
1 No cyanosis at rest.
2 Auscultation. Long pulmonary ejection murmur and even a thrill (considerable pulmonary blood flow).
3 Chest X-ray. Lung fields virtually normal.

TREATMENT
The prognosis in the acyanotic patient is reasonably good without surgery. However, there remains the risk of paradoxical embolism and cerebral abscess and the mortality of surgery is lower than for cyanotic Fallot's Tetralogy. Total correction is therefore advised.

Pulmonary atresia

ANATOMY
There is complete obstruction at the pulmonary valve or in the main

G

pulmonary artery. Pulmonary blood flow is maintained by blood flow from bronchial arteries.

CLINICAL PRESENTATION

As in the most severe forms of Fallot's Tetralogy except for:

1 Auscultation—no pulmonary ejection murmur but a soft continuous murmur produced by bronchial arterial collateral flow or by a persistent ductus arteriosus. The continuous murmur may be loudest below the clavicles or at the back.

2 Chest X-ray. As in Fallot's Tetralogy except that the lung fields show a mottled, lace-like pattern (enlarged bronchial arteries).

3 Cardiac catheterization and angiography. The pulmonary artery cannot be entered with the catheter and injection of contrast medium into the right ventricle shows the aorta filling through a ventricular septal defect and no filling of the pulmonary artery.

PROGNOSIS

Most die in infancy. A few patients maintain sufficient pulmonary flow via bronchial collaterals to survive to adult life.

TREATMENT

In the type of pulmonary atresia in which the pulmonary artery has a lumen, a shunt is made from the front of the right ventricle to the pulmonary artery using an aortic homograft including the aortic valve. A Blalock operation is an alternative.

DIFFERENTIAL DIAGNOSIS OF CYANOTIC CONGENITAL HEART DISEASE AT THE BED-SIDE

Ischaemic Lung Fields

Fallot's Tetralogy

Moderate right ventricular hypertrophy and a pulmonary ejection murmur.

Pulmonary valve stenosis with atrial communication

Giant *a* wave in jugular venous pulse, marked right ventricular hypertrophy on the electrocardiogram and poststenotic dilatation of the pulmonary artery on chest X-ray.

Tricuspid Atresia

The electrocardiogram shows left axis deviation (p. 44) and left ventricular hypertrophy.

Plethoric Lung Fields

Transposition of the great arteries
Right ventricular hypertrophy and narrow vascular pedicle on chest X-ray.

Persistent truncus arteriosus
Left ventricular hypertrophy and no pulmonary artery on chest X-ray.

Eisenmenger situation
Marked right ventricular hypertrophy, palpable P$_2$ and large main pulmonary arteries with translucent peripheral lung fields on chest X-ray.

Total anomalous pulmonary venous drainage
Right ventricular hypertrophy, large pulmonary artery and *cottage loaf* appearance on the chest X-ray.

PULMONARY ARTERY STENOSIS

Types (Fig. 9.10)

Type I   Single constriction of the main trunk or right or left pulmonary artery.
Type II   Stenosis at the bifurcation of the main pulmonary trunk.
Type III   Multiple peripheral stenoses.
Type IV   Combination of types I and III.

Haemodynamics

Systolic pressure in pulmonary artery is raised but not the diastolic pressure. Often associated with other congenital abnormalities, e.g. the rubella syndrome, supravalve aortic stenosis.

Clinical

As in pulmonary valve stenosis except:

Auscultation
No ejection click (valve not affected).
Systolic or continuous murmur heard widely in thorax.
Pulmonary component of second sound normal or loud (raised

systolic pressure above valve) and is normally split and moves with respiration.

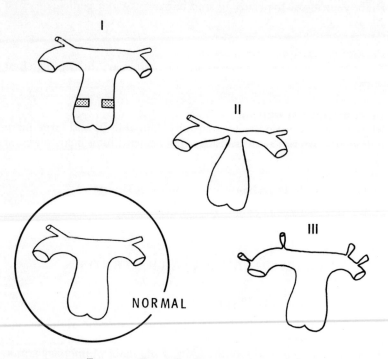

FIG. 9.10   Types of pulmonary artery stenosis

Cardiac catheterization
Pressure gradient in pulmonary artery.

Angiography
Site delineated.

Prognosis

Stenotic orifice tends to grow with age and lesion is therefore not progressive. If central and severe, requires relief of obstruction.

Treatment

Patch across central stenosis.

PULMONARY REGURGITATION

Aetiology

1   Pulmonary hypertension—Severe pulmonary hypertension from any cause causes dilatation of the main pulmonary artery and the pulmonary valve ring. Pulmonary valve regurgitation is frequent in all types of pulmonary hypertension.
2   Following pulmonary valvotomy.
3   Congenital absence of pulmonary valve.
4   Bacterial endocarditis involving the pulmonary valve.

Haemodynamics

The regurgitant flow is not gross in a pulmonary hypertensive patient and by itself scarcely influences the course of the disease.

Pulmonary valve lesions causing severe regurgitation undoubtedly increase the volume load of the right ventricle. The heart enlarges and the right ventricular volume and systolic pressure rise, but the diastolic pressure is little changed and effort tolerance is normal.

Clinical Presentation

Symptoms
None from the pulmonary regurgitation. Symptoms are those associated with the disease responsible for the regurgitation.

Signs
High-pitched, blowing early diastolic murmur in the pulmonary area and down the left sternal edge—indistinguishable on auscultation from the murmur of aortic regurgitation.

Differentiation of Pulmonary from Aortic Regurgitation

1   Water hammer pulse indicates aortic regurgitation.
2   Clinical evidence of pulmonary hypertension (p. 84) makes pulmonary regurgitation a possible diagnosis.
3   In the absence of peripheral signs of aortic regurgitation or of signs of pulmonary hypertension, the murmur is practically always a result of mild aortic regurgitation.

Prognosis

Pulmonary regurgitation does not appreciably alter the prognosis of pulmonary hypertensive disease. Post-operative pulmonary re-gurgitation is associated with some cardiac enlargement, but usually does not influence the relief of symptoms obtained from cardiac surgery in Fallot's Tetralogy or pulmonary valve stenosis.

Treatment

Relief of pulmonary hypertension, when possible, abolishes the leak. No direct operation for pulmonary regurgitation itself is indicated.

CHAPTER 10
TRICUSPID VALVE DISEASE

TRICUSPID STENOSIS

Aetiology

Almost all cases of tricuspid stenosis are rheumatic in origin, with coincident damage to the mitral valve. Five per cent of patients with mitral stenosis undergoing mitral valvotomy have some degree of associated rheumatic tricuspid stenosis.

Rare causes of tricuspid stenosis include carcinoid tumours, systemic lupus erythematosus and congenital tricuspid stenosis.

Pathology

The end result of rheumatic endocarditis of the tricuspid valve is a roundish hole in a diaphragm composed of fused tricuspid leaflets. Some degree of incompetence is therefore also the rule. The right atrium is dilated and hypertrophied.

Haemodynamics

Narrowing of the triscuspid valve has two effects on the circulation:
1 The right atrial pressure is abnormally high—a high pressure is required to maintain blood flow through the valve.
2 The cardiac output is low because of the increased resistance to blood flow through the tricuspid valve.

Clinical Presentation

Symptoms
1 High right atrial pressure transmitted to the superior and inferior venae cavae causes unpleasant throbbing in the head on stooping: throbbing pulsation in the neck; abdominal discomfort (distended liver).
2 Low cardiac output is responsible for fatigue and ankle swelling. Dyspnoea, when present, is mainly attributable to associated mitral valve disease.

Clinical examination

GENERAL
Cyanotic tinge to cheeks.

JUGULAR VENOUS PRESSURE
1   The venous pressure is abnormally high.
2   Powerful right atrial contraction causes a dominant *a* wave in patients who remain in sinus rhythm.
3   The right atrial pressure falls slowly during ventricular diastole as the obstructed atrium gradually empties into the right ventricle. The *y* descent of the jugular venous pulse is characteristically slow and gentle.

AUSCULTATION
1   A diastolic murmur maximal in the tricuspid area, accentuated during inspiration (turbulent flow across the tricuspid valve in diastole). Presystolic accentuation of the murmur is present in the few patients who remain in sinus rhythm.
2   A pansystolic murmur is usually present (associated tricuspid incompetence being the rule).
3   A tricuspid opening snap, similar to a mitral opening snap, is occasionally heard immediately before the diastolic murmur.

Electrocardiogram

P waves taller than 2·5 mm (the P pulmonale of right atrial hypertrophy). A P mitrale is also present when the left atrium is enlarged due to mitral valve disease.

No P waves are seen, of course, if the rhythm is atrial fibrillation.

Chest X-ray

Prominent right heart border of an enlarged right atrium.

Cardiac catheterization

End-diastolic gradient across tricuspid valve (usually small).

Treatment

Medical

Reduction of physical exertion to a minimum and administration of diuretics may control the symptoms produced by fluid retention, but medical management of the severe case is unsatisfactory.

Surgery

Tricuspid valvotomy, either closed or under direct vision, produces tricuspid regurgitation because the diaphragmatic valve splits without relation to the chordal attachments and leaves unsupported cusps. Valve replacement is the only effective surgical measure and is indicated if the symptoms cannot be controlled by medical treatment.

TRICUSPID REGURGITATION

Aetiology

Tricuspid regurgitation may be functional (no disease of the tricuspid valve leaflets) or organic.

Functional tricuspid regurgitation
Any dilatation of the right ventricle may involve the tricuspid ring rendering the tricuspid valve regurgitant. Functional tricuspid regurgitation is therefore the result of right ventricular failure, particularly when atrial fibrillation is present, as this rhythm increases right ventricular dilatation.

Organic tricuspid regurgitation

RHEUMATIC
The cusps are fibrotic and deformed and there is shortening with some fusion of the chordae tendineae. Usually some fusion of the tricuspid leaflets has also occurred during the acute rheumatic process, and there are signs of tricuspid stenosis in addition to those of tricuspid regurgitation. Rheumatic mitral valve disease is practically always present.

CONGENITAL
Ebstein's disease (p. 241); endocardial cushion defects (p. 193).

BACTERIAL ENDOCARDITIS
Particularly in 'mainlining' drug addicts.

Haemodynamics

The regurgitant valve allows blood to flow into the right atrium during ventricular systole. During diastole the right ventricle receives this blood in addition to that reaching the right atrium from the great veins, so that the right atrium and right ventricle have an increased volume load and become dilated and hypertrophied.

Clinical Presentation
Symptoms
From increased venous pressure and low cardiac output (see tricuspid stenosis).

Clinical examination

JUGULAR VENOUS PRESSURE
The venous pressure is high. Regurgitation of blood into the right atrium during ventricular systole often causes a brisk rise in right atrial pressure and is responsible for a tall *v* wave. The *y* descent, in the absence of tricuspid stenosis, is normal, i.e. steep. Hepatic pulsation occurs synchronously with the *v* wave.

CARDIAC IMPULSES
Forceful movement at the left sternal edge produced by right ventricular hypertrophy and dilatation.

AUSCULTATION
Pansystolic murmur maximal at the lower end of the sternum becoming louder with inspiration (turbulence of the regurgitant jet).

LIVER
Systolic pulsation.

Electrocardiogram
Usually atrial fibrillation with right ventricular hypertrophy.

Chest X-ray
Increased transverse diameter of the heart (enlarged right atrium and ventricle). Prominence of the right cardiac border (enlarged right atrium).

Cardiac catheterization and angiography
Injection of contrast into the right ventricle shows regurgitation and may outline thickened valve cusps.

Prognosis

Control of the heart rate with digitalis and treatment of right ventricular failure along the usual lines will abolish the signs of tricuspid regurgitation when this is functional and due purely to stretching of the tricuspid ring. The prognosis then depends on the cause of the right ventricular failure.

Severe organic tricuspid regurgitation causes prolonged disabling symptoms from congestive failure and a high venous pressure.

Treatment

Medical treatment
This includes rest, digitalis and diuretics to improve the function of the right ventricle, and may control the more severe symptoms.

Surgery

INDICATIONS
When tricuspid regurgitation is organic it is usual to repair or replace the valve at the time of operation on the mitral valve. Functional tricuspid regurgitation is best left to resolve subsequently.

TECHNIQUES

Tricuspid valvoplasty
For normal cusps. Plication of the valve ring reduces the size of the orifice and allows the cusps to become competent but long term results of valvoplasty are disappointing. A split septal cusp is sutured during correction of an endocardial cushion defect.

Tricuspid valve replacement
When the cusps are deformed, plication fails to cure the regurgitation and the valve is therefore replaced with a prosthesis. A low profile disc prosthesis is used in order not to encroach on the right ventricular cavity.

RESULTS
The correction of severe tricuspid regurgitation during the operation for correction of mitral valve disease improves the prognosis of operation by increasing forward flow in the post-operative period.

CHAPTER 11
LEFT TO RIGHT SHUNTS

Mechanism

The resistance to blood flow through normal pulmonary vessels is much less than the resistance offered by the systemic arterioles, and the pressures in the right ventricle and pulmonary artery are therefore proportionately lower than those in the left ventricle and aorta. A communication between the left and right sides of the heart results in blood flowing through the defect from left to right due to this pressure difference.

Sites

Communications usually occur between corresponding parts of the heart, i.e. between the atria, the ventricles or between the aorta and pulmonary artery. Occasionally defects connect different levels e.g. from left ventricle to right atrium or from aorta to right atrium.

Haemodynamics

Blood flows across the defect, through the lungs, back to the heart and across the defect again. This useless circular flow of already oxygenated blood is termed the left to right shunt which has to be accommodated by the heart in addition to the normal venous return and cardiac output. All cardiac chambers and great vessels through which the shunt flows dilate, and the appropriate ventricle hypertrophies to compensate for it. An atrial septal defect causes a volume overload of the right ventricle, a persistent ductus arteriosus of the left ventricle and a ventricular septal defect overloads both ventricles (Figs. 11.4, 11.13, 11.9).

Magnitude of the Shunt

Depends on:
1 The size of the defect.
2 The pressure difference across the defect. The pressures in the right side of the heart may be raised by the presence of pulmonary stenosis or a raised pulmonary vascular resistance, which will reduce the shunt.

Complications of Left to Right Shunts

Cardiac failure
Volume overload of the involved ventricle.

Bacterial endocarditis
Turbulence at the site of the defect.

Raised pulmonary vascular resistance
A number of patients react, for no known reason, to large left to right shunts by intimal thickening and medial hypertrophy of the small pulmonary arteries, which raises the resistance to the flow of blood through the lungs.

EMBRYOLOGY OF THE HEART

Early Development

Bilateral straight tubes fuse with septum disappearing
(Fig. 11.1a and b)
Endocardial tubes develop in the cardiogenic plate and are surrounded by the myoepicardial mantle. Constrictions mark off the chambers—truncus arteriosus, bulbus cordis, ventricle, atrium and sinus venosus (Fig. 11.1a).

The single tube twists to the left and loses its symmetry
The heart then falls into the pericardial cavity, the dorsal mesentery breaking down to form the transverse sinus (Fig. 11.1c).

Development of endocardial cushions and venous valves
Dorsal and ventral endocardial cushions form between atrium and ventricle narrowing the atrioventricular orifice and forming the A–V valves (Fig. 11.1d). The right part of the sinus venosus receives most of the venous blood via the ductus venosus through the right side of the liver, and becomes absorbed into the atrium.

The pulmonary veins drain into the left part of the sinus venosus which also becomes absorbed into the atrium.

Bulbus cordis
The bulbo-ventricular ridge between bulbus and ventricle disappears, incorporating the bulbus into the ventricle (Fig. 11.1e). Longitudinal spiral endocardial cushions form in the truncus arteriosus and bulbus and fuse to form a spiral septum, which cuts

off the aorta from the pulmonary artery distally and proximally divides the infundibulum of the right ventricle from the vestibule of the left (Fig. 12.6). For further development of atrial septum, ventricular septum, bulbus, truncus and aortic arches, see pp. 193, 201, 232, 249.

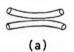

(a)

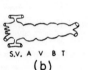

S.V. A V B T
(b)

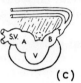

(c)

Pair of endocardial tubes

Tubes fuse and form constrictions

Heart falls into pericardium

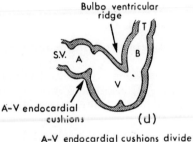

Bulbo ventricular ridge

A-V endocardial cushions

(d)

A-V endocardial cushions divide atrium from ventricle

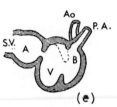

(e)

Bulbus (infundibulum of right ventricle, vestibule of left) incorporated into ventricle

Fig. 11.1   Early development of the heart

ATRIAL SEPTAL DEFECTS

Embryology

1 The sickle-shaped septum primum grows down to the atrioventricular endocardial cushions, leaving initially a gap, the ostium primum, between its lower margin and the cushions (Fig. 11.2).

2 The septum primum reaches the A–V endocardial cushions obliterating the ostium primum, and the upper part of the septum breaks down to form the ostium secundum (Fig. 11.2).

3 The septum secundum grows down on the right side of the septum primum, leaving a communication between right and left

atria, the foramen ovale. Oxygenated umbilical vein blood enters from the inferior vena cava and is diverted by the valve of the IVC through the foramen ovale into the left atrium (Fig. 11.2).

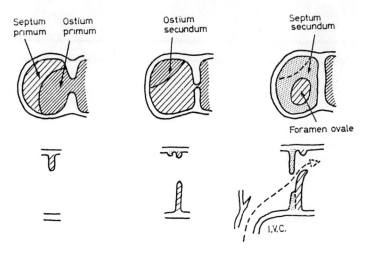

FIG. 11.2   Development of atrial septum

4   Abnormalities of absorption of the sinus venosus and pulmonary veins into the atrium may result in anomalous connections of pulmonary veins to the right atrium.

Types of Atrial Septal Defect (Fig. 11.3)

Secundum defects (90%)
Persistence of the ostium secundum due to failure of the septum secundum to develop normally results in a defect which lies behind the coronary sinus and does not reach the A–V valves.

Sinus venosus defects (5%)
Failure of proper absorption of the sinus venosus into the right atrium results in a high atrial septal defect with anomalous connections of the right upper and middle lobe pulmonary veins into the superior vena cava.

Endocardial cushion defects (5%)
Failure of the septum primum and the two endocardial cushions to meet in the centre of the heart results in defects of varying severity:

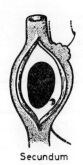 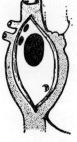 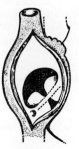

Secundum   Sinus venosus   Endocardial cushion

FIG. 11.3   Types of atrial septal defect

OSTIUM PRIMUM DEFECT ALONE—RARE
The defect is in front of the coronary sinus immediately above the mitral and tricuspid valves.

OSTIUM PRIMUM DEFECT AND CLEFT MITRAL VALVE
The aortic leaflet of the mitral valve is cleft in two, with abnormal chordae tendineae binding the edges of the cleft to the ventricular septum and sometimes keeping the valve competent despite the cleft.

OSTIUM PRIMUM DEFECT AND CLEFT MITRAL AND TRICUSPID VALVES
The septal leaflet of the tricuspid valve is similarly cleft.

OSTIUM PRIMUM DEFECT, CLEFT A–V VALVES AND A VENTRICULAR SEPTAL DEFECT (*Atrioventricularis communis* or *complete atrioventricular canal*)
The ventricular septal defect occurs because the part of the membranous septum that is formed from the downgrowth from the endocardial cushions is missing (201).

Hemi-anomalous pulmonary venous drainage
The right pulmonary veins may drain into the right atrium in association with any type of atrial septal defect.

Haemodynamics (Fig. 11.4)

The following two principles govern the haemodynamics:

Functionally there is a common atrium
The septal defect is usually so large that the pressures in both atria are identical, i.e. functionally the situation is a common atrium.

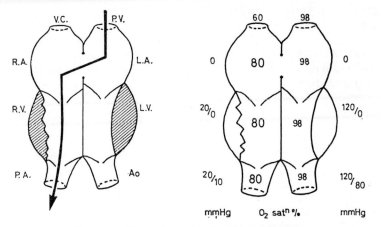

FIG. 11.4   Haemodynamics of atrial septal defect

Right ventricular filling resistance is less than the left

The shunt occurs from left to right atrium across the defect because the thin walled right ventricle poses less resistance to filling in diastole than the thicker left ventricle. This explains why no shunt occurs at birth when both ventricles are equally thick.

The shunt of oxygenated blood flows through right atrium, right ventricle, pulmonary arteries and back through pulmonary veins, left atrium and across the defect again. The right side of the heart alone is overloaded and the left ventricle is not involved (Fig. 11.4). The reduced filling pressure of the left ventricle in fact causes a smaller than normal stroke volume.

Clinical Presentation of Secundum Atrial Septal Defect

Symptoms

Usually none unless atrial fibrillation with right ventricular failure is present. This is uncommon before the age of 50.

Clinical examination

GENERAL

Normal. Occasionally signs of Marfan's syndrome are found (p. 8).

PULSE AND BLOOD PRESSURE

Pulse normal or small (reduced left ventricular output). Sinus arrhythmia disappears when the pulmonary blood flow exceeds the aortic by 3:1.

JUGULAR VENOUS PRESSURE
Normal.

CARDIAC IMPULSES
Moderate right ventricular hypertrophy of the hyperkinetic (volume overload) type.

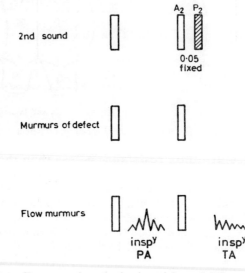

FIG. 11.5   Auscultation in atrial septal defect

AUSCULTATION

Second sound
Split to about 0·05 sec (prolongation of right ventricular systole by the volume overload and right bundle branch block) and the interval remains *fixed* during respiration (on inspiration the increased venous return enters a functionally common atrium and both ventricles receive an increased diastolic volume. Both A_2 and P_2 are delayed but the interval between them remains fixed).

Murmurs of the defect
None (a large defect without a pressure gradient across it produces no turbulence).

Flow murmurs
A pulmonary ejection systolic murmur and a diastolic tricuspid murmur are produced by the turbulence of the increased flow of the

shunt across these valves. The murmurs are louder on inspiration (increased blood flow into the heart during inspiration).

Electrocardiography
1 Right axis deviation of mean frontal QRS vector (right ventricular hypertrophy).
2 RSR pattern in lead V_1 (partial right bundle branch block from prolonged right ventricular activation).
3 Clockwise rotation of vector loop in frontal plane.

Chest X-ray
1 Pulmonary plethora (left to right shunt).
2 Enlarged right atrium, ventricular mass and pulmonary artery (increased volume in these chambers).
3 Small aorta (reduced cardiac output).

Cardiac catheterization (Fig. 11.4)
Increase in oxygen saturation in samples at atrial level (site of left to right shunt). Normal right-sided pressures unless the pulmonary vascular resistance is raised. Occasionally a *flow* gradient can be found across the pulmonary outflow due to the abnormally large flow of blood. Blood flows are difficult to assess because a true mixed venous sample cannot be obtained.

Angiography
Not routinely performed. It is difficult to obtain clear pictures of the atrial defect because of the high flow rate across it.

Differentiation of other Types of Atrial Septal Defect

Sinus venosus defect

CHEST X-RAY
Bulge at lower end of superior vena cava (site of entry of right upper and middle lobe veins).

CARDIAC CATHETERIZATION
Increase in oxygen saturation occurs at the lower end of the SVC from which pulmonary veins can be entered.

Endocardial cushion defect

GENERAL
The patient has more symptoms of dyspnoea, respiratory infections

and arrhythmias as a rule and thrives less well (mitral regurgitation).

AUSCULTATION
Pansystolic murmur of mitral regurgitation, when present, strongly suggests a cushion defect.

ELECTROCARDIOGRAPHY
1   Left axis deviation of mean frontal QRS vector (congenital abnormality of the conducting system) is present in over 90% of cases of endocardial cushion defect. V_1 shows an RSR′ pattern of 'incomplete right bundle branch block'. The vector loop is counterclockwise.
2   PR interval is prolonged more frequently than in the secundum type of defect.

CHEST X-RAY
Left atrial enlargement.

ANGIOGRAPHY
Left ventricular injection of contrast shows narrow outflow tract of left ventricle ('gooseneck') due to the anomalous aortic cusp of the mitral valve.

Hemi anomalous pulmonary venous drainage
Injection of dye into the right pulmonary artery results in a delayed appearance time at the ear compared with injection into the left pulmonary artery.

Lutembacher syndrome
(Secundum atrial septal defect with associated congenital or acquired mitral valve disease.)
    The left atrium is decompressed by the septal defect and the usual symptoms of mitral valve disease, which are due to a markedly raised left atrial pressure, do not develop. The following signs suggest its presence:

JUGULAR VENOUS PRESSURE
Raised (the pressures in both atria rise because of the mitral obstruction).

CHEST X-RAY
Large left atrium (left main bronchus elevated or left atrium visible). Calcification sometimes seen in mitral valve.

CARDIAC CATHETERIZATION
The absence of a diastolic pressure gradient across the mitral valve
does not exclude the diagnosis (the low blood flow across the valve
makes the gradient small and difficult to detect).

AT SURGERY
The only reliable diagnostic method. Unless the surgeon passes his
finger through the mitral valve during operation on every case of
atrial septal defect the diagnosis will be overlooked.

Prognosis

The patient with a moderate or large defect remains well until atrial
fibrillation occurs at the age of 45–55, after which cardiac failure
initiates a rapid downhill cause. Small defects (less than 1·5 cm in
diameter) allow a normal life span.

Failure occurs earlier in endocardial cushion defects, especially if
the pulmonary vascular resistance is increased (p. 85).

Treatment

Indications for surgery

SECUNDUM AND SINUS VENOSUS DEFECTS
Pulmonary blood flow more than twice systemic flow (indicating
that the defect is greater than 2 cm in diameter and therefore likely
to cause symptoms in later years).

ENDOCARDIAL CUSHION DEFECTS
The presence of symptoms or a large shunt (stricter indications than
for secundum defects because the results of surgery in terms of
mortality, heart block and residual mitral regurgitation are less
satisfactory).

Technique of operation

SECUNDUM DEFECTS
The defect is sutured with the assistance of cardiopulmonary bypass
(Fig. 11.6).

SINUS VENOSUS DEFECTS AND ANOMALOUS
PULMONARY VEINS
The anterior edge of the defect is sutured to the right of the anoma-
lous veins, diverting them into the left atrium (Fig. 11.6).

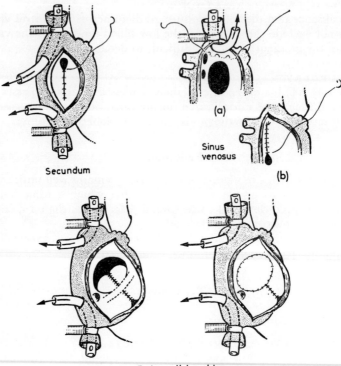

(a)

Sinus
venosus

(b)

Secundum

Endocardial cushion

FIG. 11.6   Surgery of atrial septal defects

ENDOCARDIAL CUSHION DEFECTS
The mitral and tricuspid valves are carefully repaired on cardiopulmonary bypass and the defect patched to prevent distortion of the
A–V ring (Fig. 11.6). Occasionally mitral valve replacement is
necessary.

LUTEMBACHER SYNDROME
Mitral valvotomy or valve repair is performed at the time of suture
of the septal defect.

Results

UNCOMPLICATED SECUNDUM AND SINUS VENOSUS DEFECTS
Mortality 0–2%. Morbidity is slight and is due to air embolism and
damage to the S.A. node causing atrial flutter.

SECUNDUM DEFECTS WITH ANY RISE OF PULMONARY
VASCULAR RESISTANCE
Mortality 30%.

ENDOCARDIAL CUSHION DEFECTS
Mortality 4–10%. Morbidity is significant due to heart block
(3–16%) and failure to cure mitral regurgitation, the effects of which
are aggravated by closure of the atrial defect.

VENTRICULAR SEPTAL DEFECTS

Embryology

The ventricular septum is derived from three components—the
primitive interventricular septum, an endocardial cushion downgrowth and the bulbar septum.

1 The muscular septum develops from the primitive interventricular septum (Fig. 11.7).

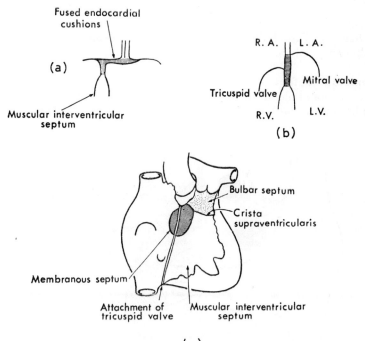

FIG. 11.7 Development of ventricular septum

2   The membranous septum is derived from a downgrowth from the right side of the A–V endocardial cushions on to the muscular septum (Fig. 11.7a). The upper part of the membranous septum separates left ventricle from right atrium when the septum straightens out because the mitral valve becomes attached higher up the septum than the tricuspid valve (Fig. 11.7b).

3   The outflow parts of the ventricles (infundibulum of the right ventricle and vestibule of the left) are separated by the proximal part of the bulbospiral septum, the distal part of which separates aorta from pulmonary artery in the truncus. The bulbar septum fuses with the membranous and muscular septa at the crista supraventricularis (Fig. 11.7c).

Types of Ventricular Septal Defect (Fig. 11.8)

Membranous ventricular septal defect
The commonest defect is a deficiency of the membranous septum immediately below the tricuspid valve. The bundle of His runs along the posterior edge of this defect.

Supracristal defect
Deficiency of the bulbar septum immediately below the aortic and pulmonary valves.

Muscular defect
One or more holes in the muscular septum. Usually they are of congenital origin but they may follow trauma or myocardial infarction.

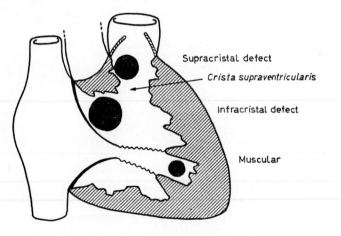

FIG. 11.8   Anatomy of ventricular septal defect

Left ventricular/right atrial defect (Gerbode defect)

Deficiency of the membranous septum above the tricuspid valve allows the left ventricle to communicate directly with the right atrium. A variant of this defect is a typical membranous defect below the tricuspid valve with a hole in the adjacent septal leaflet of the valve, which produces a similar physiological lesion.

Haemodynamics (Fig. 11.9)

Blood flows across the defect because of the pressure gradient from left to right ventricle during systole, through the pulmonary artery and veins and back through the left atrium to the left ventricle (Fig. 11.9). Both right and left ventricles have a volume overload.

Magnitude of the shunt

This depends on the following:

SIZE OF THE DEFECT

A defect less than 1 sq cm in size in the adult offers considerable resistance to blood flow from left ventricle to right ventricle, and the pulmonary blood flow is no more than twice the systemic. Large defects offer less resistance to blood flow out of the left ventricle. The pulmonary flow can be great in these cases with high pulmonary artery pressures due to the flow.

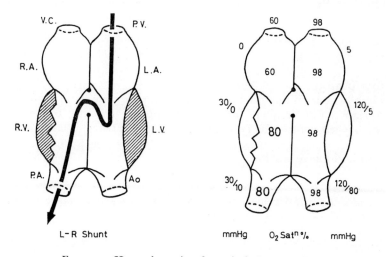

FIG. 11.9   Haemodynamics of ventricular septal defect

PULMONARY VASCULAR RESISTANCE (p. 63)

The pulmonary vascular resistance is normal when the defect is small. When the defect is large the pulmonary vascular resistance may be normal, in which case the shunt is considerable. Intimal thickening and medial hypertrophy of the pulmonary arterioles occur in some patients and increase the resistance to blood flow from right ventricle into the lungs which limits the magnitude of the left to right shunt through the defect.

Haemodynamic varieties of ventricular septal defects

1 Small defect with small shunt and normal pulmonary vascular resistance (Maladie de Roger).

2 Large defect with normal pulmonary vascular resistance and very large left to right shunt.

3 Large defect with elevated pulmonary vascular resistance, the left to right shunt being small and pulmonary arterial pressure high (p. 215).

4 Large defect with pulmonary vascular resistance greater than systemic resistance. Blood flows across the defect in a reversed direction from right to left (Eisenmenger complex p. 85).

5 Single ventricle. Commonly associated with transposition of the great vessels, dextrocardia or laevocardia. There is often a rudimentary outflow chamber below the aortic or pulmonary valve (see p. 226).

Clinical Presentation of Defects with a Normal Pulmonary Vascular Resistance

Acyanotic child with a harsh pansystolic murmur at the left sternal edge.

Symptoms

Usually none. If the shunt is large, the symptoms are those of any left to right shunt (frequent bronchitis, dyspnoea, failure to thrive). In infancy left ventricular failure is common if the defect is large.

Clinical examination

GENERAL

Normal or underweight. Sternum bulges forward in large defects with high pulmonary artery pressures.

PULSE

Normal.

JUGULAR VENOUS PRESSURE
Normal.

CARDIAC IMPULSES
Abrupt forceful apex beat (volume overload of left and to a lesser
extent right ventricles).

AUSCULTATION (Fig. 11.10)

Murmur of the defect
Harsh pansystolic murmur in the third or fourth intercostal space at
the left sternal edge (the jet is directed forwards and to the right, at
right angles to the septum) and louder on expiration (leaking left
ventricle).

Flow murmurs
 A pulmonary ejection murmur   Increased flow across the pulmonary
valve is usually obscured by the pansystolic murmur of the defect.
 Mitral diastolic murmur   Produced by torrential flow across a normal
mitral valve and indicates that the pulmonary flow is more than
twice the systemic flow.

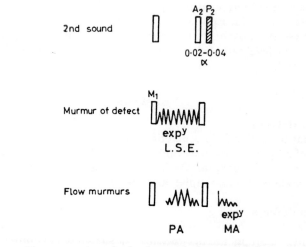

FIG. 11.10   Auscultation in ventricular septal defect

Second sound
The second sound is split (the onset of right ventricular systole is
delayed for reasons which are unknown, as there is usually no

electrocardiographic delay) and widens normally on inspiration (normal prolongation of right ventricular systole on inspiration).

Electrocardiography
Normal axis.
Voltage changes of left ventricular hypertrophy.

Chest X-ray
Pulmonary plethora (increased pulmonary blood flow). Enlargement of left atrium and ventricles.

Cardiac catheterization and angiography
1   Small defects (Fig. 11.9).
Normal pressures in right heart and pulmonary artery. Oxygen saturations of right ventricular samples may be normal if the shunt is small, and angiography, with the injection of contrast into the left ventricle, is required to demonstrate the defect.
2   Large defects.
Usually some increase in pulmonary arterial and right ventricular pressures. The magnitude of the shunt can be calculated from the rise in oxygen saturation in the right ventricle (p. 62). Angiography delineates the exact anatomy and excludes abnormalities of the great vessels, such as corrected transposition.
3   Left ventricular/right atrial (Gerbode) defects.
The increase in oxygen saturation is found at right atrial as well as ventricular level, and left ventricular injection of contrast is seen to fill the right atrium on angiocardiography.

Prognosis

Small defects
Compatible with a full normal life. Bacterial endocarditis affects one third of all patients at some time during their lives and 5% of deaths are due to this. 25% of small defects close spontaneously during childhood, as also may some large defects.

Large defects
Average life expectancy untreated is about 35 years. Large defects are often fatal in infancy because of congestive failure. If some factor limits the shunt, such as raised pulmonary vascular resistance or pulmonary stenosis, failure does not occur until middle age. Increasing infundibular hypertrophy occurs in some, converting the VSD to Fallot's Tetralogy.

Treatment

Indications for surgery

SMALL DEFECTS

Surgical closure is advised after an attack of bacterial endocarditis because further attacks are common and the myocardium may be damaged. Surgery is not performed routinely on small uncomplicated defects because the operative mortality may be higher than the risks of bacterial endocarditis and because many close spontaneously.

LARGE DEFECTS

Large defects with a pulmonary blood flow exceeding the systemic flow by more than 2:1 require closure if symptoms are present, the heart enlarged or the pulmonary artery pressure raised. In infancy the mortality of closure of the defect is higher than in older children and the pulmonary artery may be constricted by a band to limit the shunt until the infant is old enough for closure of the defect. Units skilled in infant surgery, however, are now able to close ventricular septal defects at any age with an acceptable mortality.

DEVELOPING FALLOT'S TETRALOGY

Progression to Fallot's Tetralogy with onset of cyanosis is an indication for surgery.

Technique

CLOSURE OF DEFECT

The defect is sutured (small defect) or patched (large defect) through the right atrium or a transverse incision in the right ventricle using cardiopulmonary bypass. The bundle of His running along the posterior border of the defect is carefully avoided by placing the sutures on the right side of the septum in this area.

BANDING OF PULMONARY ARTERY IN INFANCY

The artery is constricted with a coarse ligature until the pulmonary arterial pressure beyond the constriction is reduced to 30 mm Hg.

Results

CLOSURE OF SMALL DEFECTS

Low mortality (1–2%). Incidence of heart block low.

CLOSURE OF LARGE DEFECTS

Mortality
When the pulmonary vascular resistance is normal or only moderately raised (less than 8 units) the mortality is approximately 2–5%. With a markedly raised pulmonary vascular resistance (more than half systemic levels) the mortality of closure is approximately 25%.

Complete heart block
Incidence 5%. The majority of patients with permanent heart block after surgery do not survive.

Reopening of defect

BANDING OF PULMONARY ARTERY IN INFANCY
Mortality 10% (50% if a persistent ductus arteriosus is also present). Similar mortality for closure of defects in infancy in units skilled in infant surgery.

PERSISTENT DUCTUS ARTERIOSUS

Foetal Circulation

The ductus arteriosus is derived from the 6th branchial arch and connects the left pulmonary artery to the descending thoracic aorta (Fig. 13.1*b*).

Before birth
In the foetus oxygenated blood reaches the heart from the umbilical vein through the inferior vena cava. A reflexion of endocardium (the Eustachian valve of the IVC) deflects the blood towards the atrial septum and through the foramen ovale into the left atrium whence it is pumped by the left ventricle into the head, neck and arms (Fig. 11.11).

The venous return from the head streams across the right atrium into the right ventricle from which it is pumped into the pulmonary artery. The resistance of the pulmonary vasculature in the collapsed lungs is high and most of this blood passes across the ductus arteriosus to supply the lower body which is therefore supplied with blood of lower oxygen content than the head.

After birth
At birth the pulmonary vascular resistance is abruptly lowered as the lungs are inflated, and the ductus becomes obliterated within the

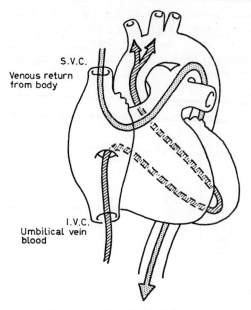

FIG. 11.11   Foetal circulation

next few hours or days. The mechanism whereby the ductus closes shortly after birth is not known—failure of this normal closure (Fig. 11.12) can be ascribed to foetal anoxia or maternal infection with rubella in some cases.

Haemodynamics of Persistent Ductus Arteriosus

Blood flows through the ductus into the lungs throughout the cardiac

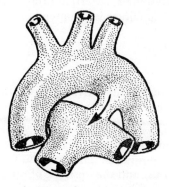

FIG. 11.12   Anatomy of persistent ductus arteriosus

cycle because the pressure in the aorta is always higher than that in the pulmonary artery (Fig. 11.13). The shunt pathway is through the pulmonary artery and lungs, left atrium, left ventricle, aorta and again through the ductus (Fig. 11.13). Only the left heart has the volume overload.

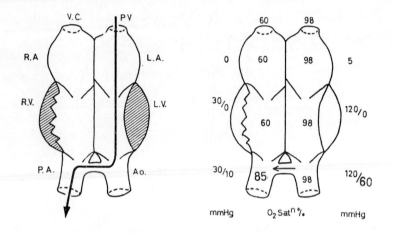

FIG. 11.13   Haemodynamics of persistent ductus̲ arteriosus

Clinical Presentation

Usually presents as an asymptomatic child with a continuous murmur in the first left intercostal space below the clavicle.

Symptoms

Usually none. If the defect is large, there may be symptoms of a large left to right shunt (dyspnoea, recurrent bronchitis, failure to thrive), and in infancy cardiac failure is common.

Clinical examination

GENERAL
Normal appearance unless the ductus is part of the rubella syndrome (mental deficiency, microcephaly, cataracts and deafness).

PULSE AND BLOOD PRESSURE
Normal when the ductus is small. A large amplitude, water-hammer pulse indicates a large ductus. The diastolic pressure is low (blood leaking from the aorta) and the upstroke of the pulse is sharp (large volume of blood ejected into an empty aorta).

JUGULAR VENOUS PRESSURE
Normal (no right sided strain).

CARDIAC IMPULSES
Abrupt forceful apex beat (left ventricle dilated and hypertrophied ejecting an abnormally large volume).

AUSCULTATION (Fig. 11.14)

Murmur of the defect
Continuous murmur, maximal in the first left intercostal space and loudest towards the end of systole and on expiration (blood flows through the ductus throughout the cardiac cycle. Towards the end of systole and during expiration the difference in pressures between aorta and pulmonary artery is at its highest level).

Flow murmurs
1   Mid-diastolic flow murmur at the apex (indicates a large ductus

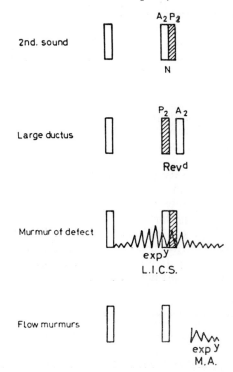

FIG. 11.14   Auscultation in persistent ductus arteriosus

H

with the increased blood flow sufficient to cause a murmur as it flows across normal mitral valve cusps in diastole).

2 Aortic ejection murmur (increased flow across the aortic valve). Usually obscured by continuous murmur.

Second sound

1 Small ductus (0–4 mm in diameter). Normal second sound.

2 Moderate ductus (5–10 mm in diameter). Single second sound (left ventricular volume overload prolongs systole, and closure of the aortic valve follows immediately after pulmonary valve closure but so close to it as to sound single. On inspiration P_2 moves across A_2 as right ventricular systole is prolonged by the normal increase in right sided flow, but is never separated from it enough to make an appreciably separate sound).

3 Large ductus (>10 mm in diameter). Reversed splitting of the second sound (left ventricular volume overload prolongs left ventricular systole so much that aortic closure falls appreciably after pulmonary closure during expiration. On inspiration P_2 moves onto A_2 and the sound becomes single—the opposite from normal).

Electrocardiography

Normal, or left ventricular hypertrophy (depending on the degree of left ventricular volume overload).

Chest X-ray

Enlargement of pulmonary artery, lung vessels, left atrium, ventricular mass, ascending aorta and knuckle (increased flow of the left to right shunt through these chambers).

Cardiac catheterization (Fig. 11.13)

A cardiac catheter can usually be passed from the pulmonary artery through the ductus into the descending aorta particularly if catheterization has been performed from a leg vein. The level of oxygen saturation rises in the pulmonary artery. The clinical signs are usually so characteristic that this step is often omitted, but 2% of patients with a typical murmur will turn out to have an aortopulmonary window and not a ductus.

Angiocardiography

Injection of contrast medium into the aorta in the region of the ductus is a reliable method for making the diagnosis. Indications for aortography are:

1 Unusual clinical features making the diagnosis uncertain.

2 Presence of other cardiac lesions which may obscure the presence

of a ductus e.g. ventricular septal defect with a high pulmonary arterial pressure.

Prognosis

Small ductus
Subacute bacterial endarteritis is the main risk (10% of all cases, 20% of whom die from the infection).

Large ductus
Life expectancy below average. Complications are:
1 Left ventricular failure and death, usually in infancy but occurring also in adult life, from the effects of prolonged left ventricular overload.
2 Bacterial endarteritis.
3 Raised pulmonary vascular resistance (p. 214).

Treatment

Indications for surgery
All patients with an uncomplicated persistent ductus, because the mortality of surgery is 0·5% which is less that for subacute bacterial endarteritis (2%).

Technique

SMALL DUCTUS
Ligation with two heavy (e.g. floss silk) ligatures and transfixion between or division between clamps and suture of the divided ends (Fig. 11.15). Recanalization is not uncommon after ligation with fine ligatures but is extremely rare following the use of floss silk as described.

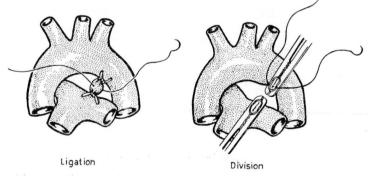

Ligation   Division

FIG. 11.15   Surgery of persistent ductus arteriosus

LARGE DUCTUS
Division and suture (ligatures cut through) (Fig. 11.15).

Results
1 Mortality 0·5%.
2 Morbidity.
   (i) Recanalization (highest after surgery for an infected ductus).
   (ii) Damage to recurrent laryngeal nerve.

RAISED PULMONARY VASCULAR RESISTANCE IN LEFT TO RIGHT SHUNTS

The resistance to blood flow through normal lungs is ten times less than the systemic arterial resistance. While many patients with large left to right intracardiac shunts have a normal pulmonary vascular resistance, in some the resistance is moderately increased and in a few it is equal to or greater than the systemic resistance.

Pathology

Changes in pulmonary arterioles
The lumen of the pulmonary arteriole becomes narrowed by intimal thickening and medial hypertrophy and may finally become obliterated by thrombosis.

Mechanism
The mechanism that causes this pathological change is unknown and there appears no obvious reason why it should affect one patient rather than another.

It is associated with large defects only and the mechanism may be different in ventricular septal defect and persistent ductus arteriosus in which the shunt is present from birth, than in secundum atrial septal defect in which a shunt cannot begin until normal involution of right ventricular hypertrophy reduces the resistance to filling of that chamber below that of the left ventricle (p. 195).

Persistence of the foetal pulmonary arteriolar pattern, which keeps the vascular resistance above systemic levels before birth, has been postulated as the cause of the high resistance in the first two defects.

Progression of the Changes

Evidence is conflicting on the subject of whether the pulmonary vascular resistance changes significantly after infancy in left to right shunts. A high resistance may persist or even increase after surgical correction of the defect.

Pulmonary Vascular Resistance Below Systemic Levels

Haemodynamics
A raised pulmonary vascular resistance alters the clinical picture of each defect by increasing the right-sided pressures (pulmonary arterial, right ventricular and right atrial), and thereby reducing the left to right shunt.

Effect on clinical presentation of individual defects
In addition to the symptoms and physical signs of the individual defects, the effects of a raised pulmonary vascular resistance modify the clinical picture:

CLINICAL EXAMINATION

General
Abnormal rounding of thoracic cage (combined effect of an increased pulmonary blood flow and an increased pulmonary vascular resistance).

Jugular venous pressure
Prominent *a* wave (right atrial hypertrophy from the increased work load on the right side of the heart).

Cardiac impulses
Right ventricular hypertrophy and palpable pulmonary valve closure (raised pressures in right ventricle and pulmonary artery). The left ventricular impulse is quieter and less bounding (the left to right shunt is reduced by the increased pulmonary resistance).

Auscultation
Loud pulmonary second sound (raised pulmonary artery pressure). The murmurs from the defect and flow murmurs are less prominent (smaller left to right shunt).

ELECTROCARDIOGRAPHY
Right ventricular hypertrophy appears or becomes more marked.

CHEST X-RAY
1   Main pulmonary artery large (effect of high pressure).

2   Peripheral lung fields translucent (narrowed small pulmonary vessels).

3   Heart size normal (volume of shunt smaller).

CARDIAC CATHETERIZATION

The pulmonary arterial pressure is increased out of proportion to the flow through the lungs. Calculation of the pulmonary vascular resistance (p. 63) shows it to be raised.

Effect on the prognosis of the defect

The association of a raised pulmonary vascular resistance with large ventricular septal defects does not appreciably alter their prognosis which is approximately 35 years, but it can be expected to worsen the prognosis of atrial septal defects and persistent ductus arteriosus.

Effect on results of surgical correction of the septal defects

A pulmonary vascular resistance greater than half the systemic level (i.e. more than 8 units) raises the surgical mortality to 20–30%. The patients die from pulmonary complications and low cardiac output in the post-operative period.

The Eisenmenger Syndrome

Definition

1   The Eisenmenger complex, as described by Eisenmenger, consists of a large ventricular septal defect with systemic levels of pulmonary vascular resistance. Under these conditions the blood flow through the defect is mainly from right to left ventricle.

2   The Eisenmenger syndrome is an extension of the term to include any connection between the two sides of the heart (at atrial, ventricular or aorto-pulmonary level) in which the pulmonary vascular resistance is at or above systemic level.

Haemodynamics

REVERSED OR BALANCED SHUNT

When the resistance in the pulmonary circulation is greater than, or the same as, that in the systemic circulation, blood flows across the defect from right to left (reversed shunt), or in both directions due to transient differences in pressure at different phases of the cardiac cycle (bi-directional, balanced shunt). There are no murmurs caused by the defect because it is large and blood flow across it is small.

CYANOSIS

The patient is centrally cyanosed except in persistent ductus arteriosus where the feet are more blue than the hands (differential cyanosis).

STRAIN ON THE HEART

The pulmonary artery and valve ring dilate with the high pressure, making the cusps regurgitant. The right ventricle and right atrium hypertrophy to maintain the high pressure.

LOW CARDIAC OUTPUT

The cardiac output falls because of the obstruction in the lungs. Right ventricular failure eventually appears.

Clinical presentation

Cyanosed patient with signs of pulmonary hypertension.

SYMPTOMS

1 Dyspnoea (effect of desaturated arterial blood on the aortic and carotid chemoreceptors). Breathlessness is least marked in the Eisenmenger persistent ductus because the desaturated blood is shunted preferentially to the lower body.
2 Angina pectoris and syncope on exertion (low cardiac output).
3 Haemoptysis (pulmonary infarction).
4 Oedema (right ventricular failure).
5 Cyanosis is often present from infancy except in atrial septal defect when the high pulmonary vascular resistance usually develops late.

CLINICAL EXAMINATION

General Central cyanosis and clubbing (right to left shunt) or differential cyanosis.

Pulse Small (low cardiac output). Atrial fibrillation appears late in the course of the disease (average age 35).

Jugular venous pressure Moderately raised with dominant *a* wave (right ventricular hypertrophy increases its filling resistance).

Cardiac impulses Right ventricular hypertrophy and palpable pulmonary valve closure (systemic pressures in right ventricle and pulmonary artery).

Auscultation As there is a small flow across a large defect there is no murmur associated with it and no flow murmurs i.e. the signs are those of pulmonary hypertension only (Fig. 11.16):

1 Right atrial fourth sound (right atrial hypertrophy).
2 Pulmonary ejection click and murmur (dilated pulmonary artery).

3 Loud pulmonary second sound (high pressure closing the valve forcibly).

4 A regurgitant diastolic murmur down the left sternal edge (pulmonary regurgitation).

5 Perhaps a pansystolic murmur in the tricuspid area (functional tricuspid regurgitation due to dilatation of the tricuspid ring with right ventricular failure).

ELECTROCARDIOGRAPHY

P pulmonale (right atrial hypertrophy) with QRS and T changes of right ventricular hypertrophy (p. 45).

CHEST X-RAY

Large proximal pulmonary arteries (high pressure) and ischaemic peripheral vessels (narrowed small arteries). Large right atrium.

CARDIAC CATHETERIZATION

1 Pulmonary artery pressure equal to systemic arterial pressure.

2 Small left to right shunt often found at the level of the defect in addition to demonstration of a right to left shunt by dye dilution studies.

ANGIOGRAPHY

Selective injection of contrast medium into the appropriate cavity may show the defect but carries an appreciable risk in these patients.

Differentiation of the site of the defect (Fig. 11.16)

It is difficult to determine the site of the defect unless the cardiac catheter crosses it or angiography is performed. One of the best clinical indications is the behaviour of the second sound:

ATRIAL SEPTAL DEFECT

Wide fixed split (the atrium is still haemodynamically a common chamber and the increased flow on inspiration prolongs the ejection time of both ventricles, maintaining their relationship with each other). Cyanosis often does not appear until adult life.

VENTRICULAR SEPTAL DEFECT

Single second sound (equal pressures in the ventricles with a large communication makes them haemodynamically a common chamber with equal ejection times. Both aortic and pulmonary valve closure occur together).

PERSISTENT DUCTUS ARTERIOSUS
Normally moving second sound (the increased inflow of blood on inspiration flows through the right ventricle in the normal way prolonging its ejection time). Differential cyanosis is pathognomonic.

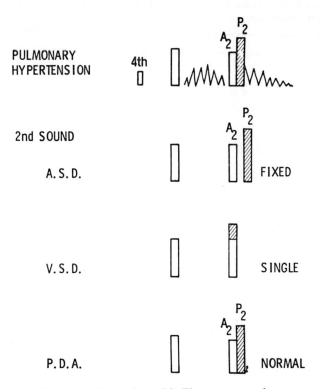

FIG. 11.16   Behaviour of second sound in Eisenmenger syndrome

Prognosis

The average age of death is 36 years. Death occurs from haemoptysis in one third of cases (pulmonary infarction with high pulmonary artery pressures), ill advised surgery, congestive cardiac failure and ventricular fibrillation. Bacterial endocarditis and cerebral abscess are less common.

Treatment

No specific treatment is available for lowering the pulmonary vascular resistance. Surgical closure of the defect is usually fatal and no benefit can be expected even if the patient survives because the symptoms and prognosis are influenced by the pulmonary resistance and not by the presence of a defect which no longer has a significant flow across it.

No treatment is necessary until complications, such as heart failure, arise. Anticoagulants are best avoided because of the incidence of dangerous haemoptyses.

OTHER LEFT TO RIGHT SHUNTS

The rarer types of left to right shunt are considered in Chapter 12 under other congenital cardiac lesions; aorto-pulmonary window on p. 235, persistent truncus arteriosus on p. 232, double outlet right ventricle on p. 230, sinus of valsalva aneurysm on p. 237 and single ventricle on p. 226.

CHAPTER 12
OTHER CONGENITAL CARDIAC LESIONS

TRANSPOSITION OF THE GREAT ARTERIES

Transposition of the great arteries is present when the aorta lies in front of the pulmonary artery. Every possible combination of inversion of ventricles or atria may bring venous or oxygenated blood into the aorta but only two combinations are of numerical significance—so called 'simple' or dextro-transposition (Fig. 12.1B) and 'corrected' or laevo-transposition (Fig. 12.1C).

Simple (Dextro-) Transposition

Embryology

The primitive heart loop has fallen to the right into the pericardial cavity in the normal way (Fig. 12.2) but maldevelopment of the spiral septum in the truncus arteriosus, with or without poor growth of the right ventricular infundibular region, causes the aorta to arise anteriorly from the right ventricle and pulmonary artery to arise posteriorly from the left ventricle. The aorta itself lies to the right of the pulmonary artery.

Haemodynamics

Instead of being in series, the two circulations, pulmonary and systemic, are in parallel with venous blood circulating round the body and oxygenated blood circulating round the lungs (Fig. 12.1B). This is incompatible with life unless a communication—ductus arteriosus, ventricular or atrial septal defect—exists to allow mixing of the circulations.

Clinical presentation

1   Severely cyanosed infant in first two weeks of life.
2   No murmurs; second heart sound single.
3   ECG normal initially; right axis deviation, normal at this age, is the rule with often a small P pulmonale.
4   Chest X-ray; large heart with plethoric lung fields is highly characteristic. Plethoric lung fields alone in a cyanosed infant makes transposition highly likely.

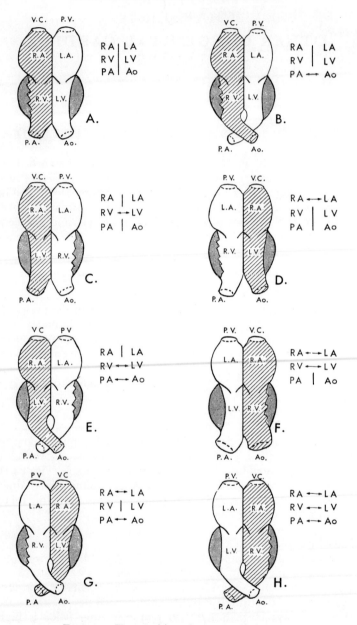

Fig. 12.1   Transposition of great arteries—types

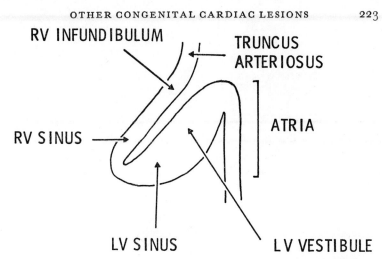

FIG. 12.2 Primitive heart loop falls to right (dextro-transposition)

5 Cardiac catheterization and angiography; delineates anatomy, site of shunts and associated anomalies.

Management

SIMPLE TRANSPOSITION

Neonate
Balloon atrioseptostomy (Rashkind). Emergency creation of an atrial septal defect is mandatory in the newborn period (70% mortality in first month of life without this operation). A catheter with a balloon at its tip is passed through the foramen ovale from the leg, inflated and drawn sharply back across the septum, splitting it and allowing the circulations to mix. Cyanosis relieved in 50–70%.

Failure of balloon atrioseptostomy to relieve cyanosis
Blalock–Hanlon operation (Fig. 12.3) making an atrial septal defect by excising the back of the septum in a clamp. Or Mustard operation as definitive operation in infancy (see below).

Within first two years
Transpose atria (Mustard operation, Fig. 12.4). Atrial septum excised and a baffle of pericardium inserted to divert pulmonary venous blood to tricuspid valve and hence aorta, leaving the systemic venous return from venae cavae to pass behind the baffle to the mitral valve and hence the pulmonary artery. Mortality 10–15%.

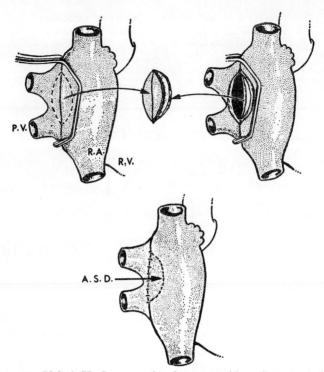

FIG. 12.3   Blalock–Hanlon operation for transposition of great arteries

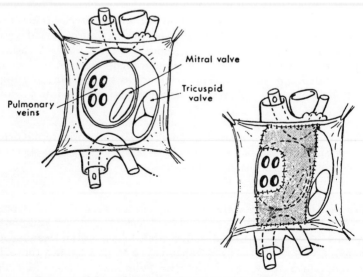

FIG. 12.4   Mustard operation for transposition of great arteries

SIMPLE TRANSPOSITION AND VSD

Balloon atrioseptostomy and band pulmonary artery to prevent excessive pulmonary blood flow if infant is in heart failure. Mustard operation later including closure of VSD.

SIMPLE TRANSPOSITION AND VSD AND PULMONARY STENOSIS

Balloon atrioseptostomy followed by Rastelli operation later (Fig. 12.12). A tunnel of cloth is sutured between the ventricular septal defect and the aorta, diverting LV blood to aorta. The pulmonary artery is ligated and divided and the distal end joined to the front of the right ventricle by a tube containing a valve.

Corrected (Laevo-) Transposition

Embryology

In corrected or laevo-transposition the primitive heart loop has fallen to the left into the pericardium, instead of to the right (Fig. 12.5). The spiral septum again develops abnormally with the aorta anterior and to the left of the pulmonary artery but this time the ventricle containing oxygenated blood lies under the aorta. This ventricle looks, however, anatomically like a right ventricle with a tricuspid valve, muscular trabecula and an infundibulum. The systemic venous return from the cavae flows through a bicuspid ('mitral') valve into a smooth walled ('left') ventricle and into the pulmonary artery.

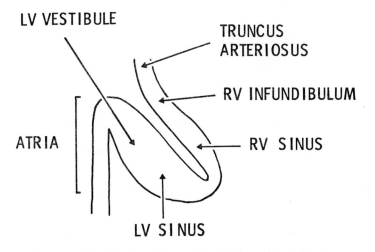

FIG. 12.5   Primitive heart loop falls to left (laevotransposition)

Haemodynamics

Although the great vessels are transposed, inversion of the ventricles has 'corrected' the physiology and the infant is not cyanosed (Fig. 12.1C). Associated defects—septal, valve stenosis etc.—occur in 80%.

Clinical presentation

1 Clinical presentation depends on associated defects.

2 Heart block is common (A–V bundles pursue a long course on right side of septum). Atrial fibrillation is also common. This condition is the most common cause of atrial fibrillation in childhood.

3 ECG may be normal or show left axis deviation.

4 Chest X-ray—abnormally narrow vascular pedicle (aortic knuckle inconspicuous and pulmonary artery over to right).

Management of corrected transposition

Does not require treatment of itself. Surgery of associated defects is avoided where possible because of the risk of producing heart block and because anomalous coronary arteries limit access to 'right' ventricle.

SINGLE VENTRICLE

Definition

A ventricular chamber receiving blood from both atrioventricular valves, or from the single atrioventricular valve. From this chamber the arterial trunks emerge with their coni (infundibulum of right ventricle, vestibule of left ventricle). One or both of these coni may be sufficiently well developed to comprise a small outlet chamber.

Classification

Classification of the various types of single ventricle depends on consideration of the interrelation of the situs, venous drainage, atria, A–V valves, dominant ventricle and great arteries.

Venous drainage

The venous drainage depends on the situs. In situs solitus (normal) the IVC is on the right. In situs inversus it is on the left. In visceral heterotaxy there is no IVC, the blood from the lower body draining via the azygos system. In addition there is a central liver and stomach, no spleen or multiple bilateral spleens.

Atria

The atria also depend on the situs. In situs solitus the morphological right atrium (fossa ovalis, crista terminalis, etc.) is on the right. In situs inversus it is on the left. In visceral heterotaxy there is usually a common atrium with the four pulmonary veins entering via a midline sump.

Atrio-ventricular valves

The number of A–V valves depends on the atria. If there are two atria there are two A–V valves. A single atrium has one A–V valve.

The number of cusps in the A–V valves depends on the situs and the loop (Figs. 12.2–12.5). The normal (D) loop with situs solitus gives a bicuspid (mitral) valve on the left and tricuspid on the right. An L loop with situs solitus gives a biscupid (mitral) valve on the right. The opposite is true of situs inversus.

Ventricles

There are four types of ventricular pattern:

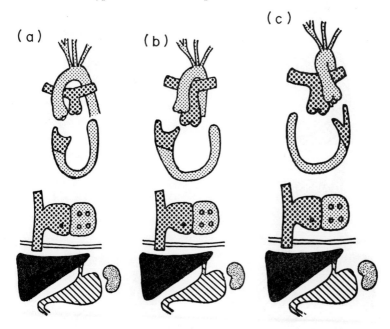

FIG. 12.6   Single ventricle type A (Absent R–V sinus). (*a*) Normally related great arteries with the small chamber to the right under the P.A. (*b*) Dextro-transposition with small chamber to the right under aorta. (*c*) Laevo-transposition with small chamber to the left under aorta (after Webb-Peploe)

TYPE A—ABSENT R–V SINUS (Fig. 12.6a, b, c)

Predominantly left ventricle (smooth walled) with a small residual chamber representing the RV infundibulum. In normally related great arteries the small chamber is to the right under the PA (Fig. 12.6a). In dextrotransposition the chamber is to the right but under the aorta (Fig. 12.6b). In laevo-transposition it is to the left and under the aorta (Fig. 12.6c). (Variant: laevotransposition with a small chamber or blind pouch).

TYPE B—ABSENCE OF BOTH LV SINUS AND
LV VESTIBULE (Fig. 12.7a, b)

The entire ventricle is right morphologically (trabeculated wall) and

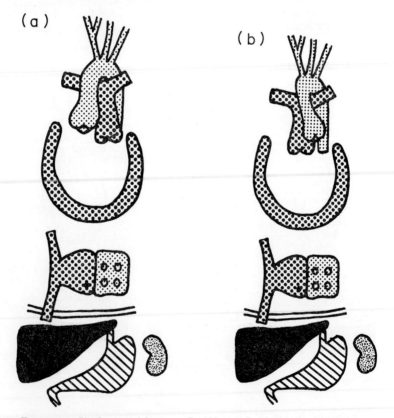

(a)   (b)

FIG. 12.7 Single ventricle type B (Absent L–V sinus). (a) Dextro-transposition with aorta to the front and right of the P.A. (b) Laevo-transposition with aorta to the front and left of the P.A. (after Webb-Peploe)

both great vessels arise from it. In dextrotransposition the aorta lies in front and to the right of the PA (Fig. 12.7*a*): in laevotransposition it lies to the front and left of the PA (Fig. 12.7*b*). Normally related great vessels have not been described with Type B.

TYPE C—INDETERMINATE VENTRICULAR MORPHOLOGY (Fig. 12.8*a*, *b*)

Occurs with all three varieties of great artery anatomy (e.g. Fig. 12.8*a*); and with visceral heterotaxy (e.g. Fig. 12.12), in which case there is almost always severe pulmonary stenosis or atresia.

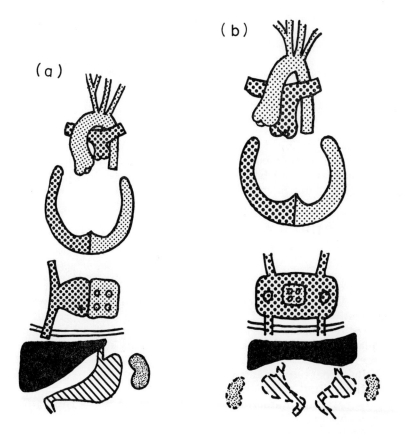

FIG. 12.8 Single ventricle type C (Indeterminate ventricular morphology). (*a*) Normal great artery relationship. (*b*) Visceral heterotaxy and dextro-transposition (after Webb-Peploe)

TYPE D—NO VENTRICULAR SINUSES

Incompatible with life. Small walnut sized heart.

Haemodynamics

Depends on degree of pulmonary stenosis, i.e. pulmonary atresia causes severe cyanosis and early death; moderate pulmonary stenosis causes slight cyanosis and minimal rise of LA pressure; no pulmonary stenosis allows a torrential pulmonary blood flow, and a high left atrial pressure, if the left atrium is not decompressed by a large ASD.

Clinical Presentation

Those with severe cyanosis are confused with Fallot's Tetralogy: those with no pulmonary stenosis with a large VSD. Differentiation is by catheterization and angiography to delineate the anatomy.

Treatment

Patients with severe pulmonary stenosis or atresia with marked cyanosis are palliated with a shunt (Blalock, Waterston, Fig. 9.9). Those with no pulmonary stenosis and a large shunt are palliated by pulmonary artery banding (p. 207). Total correction with careful placing of a large interventricular prosthetic cloth septum is possible.

DOUBLE OUTLET RIGHT VENTRICLE

Anatomical Types

Both great arteries arise from the right ventricle with a ventricular septal defect allowing left ventricular blood to reach the systemic circulation (Fig. 12.9). Pulmonary stenosis may also be present. The degree of cyanosis depends on the size and site of the ventricular septal defect and the severity of the pulmonary stenosis.

TYPE I—Ventricles normally situated.

A. Pulmonary artery anterior.

1 Infracristal (posterior, subaortic) VSD.

2 Supracristal (anterior, subpulmonary) VSD (Taussig-Bing anomaly).

B. Aorta anterior (great arteries transposed).

1 Infracristal (subpulmonary) VSD.

2 Supracristal (subaortic) VSD.

TYPE II—Ventricles inverted.

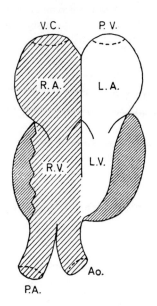

FIG. 12.9   Double outlet right ventricle

Haemodynamics and Clinical Presentation

If there is no pulmonary stenosis and the pulmonary vascular resistance is low, there is little or no cyanosis due to the large left to right shunt and the patient presents like a VSD (p. 204).

When severe pulmonary stenosis is present, the patient presents like Fallot's Tetralogy (p. 175).

When the pulmonary vascular resistance is high, the patient presents like an Eisenmenger complex (p. 216). Cyanosis also occurs when the VSD lies directly under the pulmonary artery and shunts directly into it leaving desaturated blood to enter the aorta (Types IA2 and IB1).

Clinical Diagnosis

The history of mild cyanosis or cyanosis on exertion may help to differentiate the lesion from a VSD. The larger than usual heart on the chest X-ray helps to differentiate it from Fallot's Tetralogy.

The definitive diagnosis is made at angiography:

1   The aortic and pulmonary valves are at the same transverse level.

2   The VSD is further than normal from the aortic ring.
3   Discontinuity between aortic valve ring and anterior leaflet of mitral valve—the diagnostic feature.

Treatment

On cardiopulmonary bypass a Dacron patch is used to make a tunnel from the ventricular septal defect to the aorta across the right ventricular outflow tract, separating the two circulations. Pulmonary stenosis is relieved if present. Such a patch can be seen in Fig. 12.12(3).

PERSISTENT TRUNCUS ARTERIOSUS

Embryology

Spiral endocardial ridges in the bulbus and truncus arteriosus normally join and form a spiral septum, dividing the truncus into aorta and pulmonary artery, and forming the aortic and pulmonary semilunar valves (Fig. 12.10). The bulbar septum forms the upper part of the ventricular septum, separating the infundibulum of the right ventricle from the vestibule of the left.

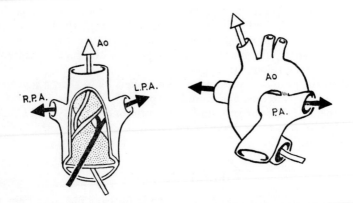

FIG. 12.10   Development of spiral bulbar septum (after Hudson, 1965)

Failure of the proximal septum to form results in one artery leaving the heart (persistent truncus), one semilunar valve (2, 3 or 4 cusps) and a deficient ventricular septum (ventricular septal defect).

Types (Fig. 12.11)

Type I
The pulmonary artery is recognizable as a separate artery (deficiency of the lower spiral septum only).

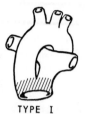

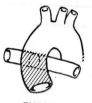

TYPE I
Lower spiral septum deficient
(pulmonary artery recognizable
as separate artery)

TYPE II
No spiral septum
(pulmonary arteries
arise together)

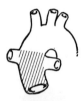

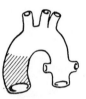

TYPE III
No spiral septum
(pulmonary arteries arise
separately)

TYPE IV
Failure of 6th arch to develop
(no ductus nor pulmonary
artery remnant)

FIG. 12.11   Persistent truncus arteriosus—types

Type II
The pulmonary arteries arise together (no spiral septum).

Type III
The pulmonary arteries arise separately (no spiral septum).

Type IV
The pulmonary arteries arise from the descending aorta (failure of 6th arch to develop, so there is no ductus nor pulmonary artery remnant).

Pseudo-truncus is a term used sometimes to describe pulmonary atresia in Fallot's Tetralogy (p. 179). A pulmonary artery remnant is always present.

Haemodynamics

Complete mixing of the circulations necessarily occurs. The oxygen
saturation of the systemic arterial blood depends on the percentage
of pulmonary venous blood in the mixture.

Low pulmonary vascular resistance

With large flow into the pulmonary artery, the mixed systemic blood
will be mainly pulmonary venous blood and little cyanosis occurs.
The left ventricle dilates to accommodate the flow.

High pulmonary vascular resistance

Usual if infancy is survived, because the shunt would otherwise be
enormous. The small or absent shunt means that the systemic arterial
blood has equal systemic and venous components and cyanosis is
marked.

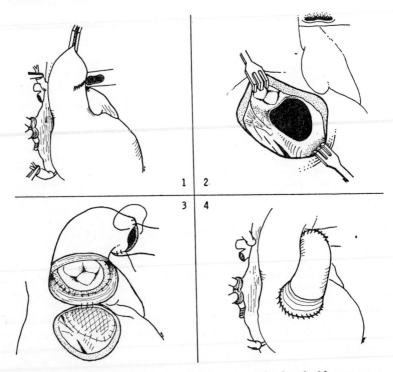

FIG. 12.12   Rastelli operation. 1   Pulmonary arteries detached from aorta.
2   Right ventricle opened showing VSD and aortic valve. 3   Patch directs
LV blood from VSD through RV to aorta: conduit containing valve
sutured between RV and pulmonary arteries. 4   Completed operation

In both types the right ventricular pressure is at systemic level and right ventricular hypertrophy occurs.

Clinical Presentation

Usually presents as an infant in heart failure with pulmonary plethora, little cyanosis and usually a single second sound.

Prognosis

Most die of congestive cardiac failure in infancy.

Treatment

1   Rastelli operation (Fig. 12.12). The ventricular septal defect is patched in such a way that left ventricular blood is diverted to the aorta. The pulmonary arteries are detached from the aorta and a tube containing an aortic homograft valve is used to connect right ventricle to pulmonary arteries.

2   Banding of pulmonary arteries. Palliative reduction of shunt.

AORTO-PULMONARY WINDOW

Embryology

Deficiency of the distal part of the spiral septum (p. 191) allows a communication between aorta and pulmonary artery above the semilunar valves, which are normal (Fig. 12.13).

Haemodynamics

As in persistent ductus arteriosus. Flow depends on the size of the communication, which is usually large and causes pulmonary hypertension.

Clinical Presentation

As persistent ductus except the following:

Auscultation

Continuous murmur is uncommon and if present suggests a co-incident ductus. The murmur is usually only systolic because of the large size of the defect and virtually equal pressures in aorta and pulmonary artery.

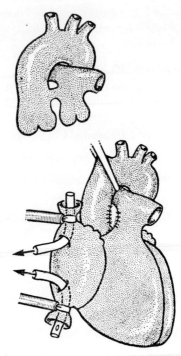

FIG. 12.13   Aorto-pulmonary window—anatomy and surgery

Cardiac catheterization
Catheter passes from pulmonary artery through the window into the ascending aorta (rather than into the descending aorta as in persistent ductus).

Aortography
Delineates lesion.

Treatment

Indications
Large shunt (small defects are not closed, unlike persistent ductus, because the operative procedure is technically more difficult and hazardous).

Technique
Using extracorporeal circulation and occlusion of the aorta, the communication is divided and both aorta and pulmonary artery sutured (Fig. 12.13), or the aorta opened and the defect patched from the inside.

SINUS OF VALSALVA ANEURYSM AND FISTULA

Anatomy (Fig. 12.14)

Aneurysms of the aortic sinuses of Valsalva develop due usually to congenital deficiency of the media between the aorta itself and the annulus fibrosus of the aortic valve. Occasionally they are mycotic or syphilitic in origin. The aneurysm projects into the adjacent cavity (right coronary sinus aneurysms bulge into the right ventricle; non-coronary sinus aneurysms bulge into the right atrium; left coronary sinus aneurysms (rare) bulge into left atrium or pericardium).

Aneurysms eventually rupture and produce a shunt from aorta to the appropriate cavity.

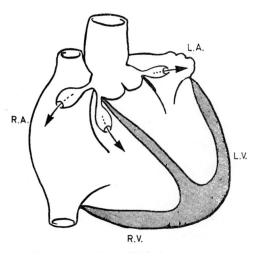

FIG. 12.14   Sinus of Valsalva aneurysms

Haemodynamics

Unruptured aneurysms cause no disturbance of cardiac function.

Rupture of an aneurysm causes a leak between aorta and relevant cavity (usually right atrium or ventricle) and the signs of a left to right shunt.

Clinical Presentation (on rupture into right heart)

The patient is normal until he suddenly develops cardiac failure and a murmur.

Symptoms
Of congestive failure (dyspnoea, oedema etc.).

Clinical examination
Continuous murmur (leaking aorta) and enlarged heart (volume overload of left to right shunt).

Cardiac catheterization and angiography
Rise in oxygen saturation of samples at right atrial or ventricular level. Aortography shows the aneurysm and the site of the rupture.

Treatment

Excision of aneurysm and suture of aorta back on to annulus using cardiopulmonary bypass.

TRICUSPID ATRESIA

Embryology

The right A–V endocardial cushion fuses to the right wall so that there is no tricuspid valve. The right ventricle is hypoplastic and there is an atrial septal defect.

Haemodynamics

An atrial septal defect allows the systemic venous return to reach the left atrium and left ventricle, and is necessary for survival. Blood enters the lungs either through a ventricular septal defect or a persistent ductus arteriosus.

Types

1 *Type I* (with normal origin of great vessels, Fig. 12.15).
Ia—pulmonary atresia and persistent ductus.
Ib—pulmonary stenosis and ventricular septal defect.
2 *Type II* (with transposition of the great vessels, Fig. 12.16).
IIa—with pulmonary stenosis.
IIb—without pulmonary stenosis.

Clinical Presentation

Usually presents as a cyanotic infant with an elevated systemic venous pressure and left axis deviation on the electrocardiogram.

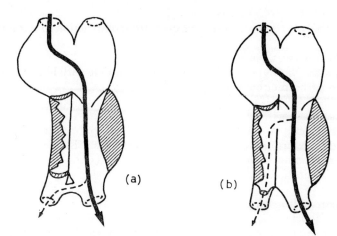

FIG. 12.15 Tricuspid atresia Type I. Great vessels arise normally.
(a) Pulmonary atresia and persistent ductus. (b) Pulmonary stenosis and
ventricular septal defect

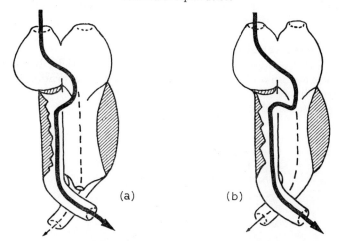

FIG. 12.16 Tricuspid atresia Type II. Transposition of great vessels.
(a) Pulmonary stenosis. (b) No pulmonary stenosis

Symptoms
Severe cyanosis, dyspnoea, syncopal attacks.

Clinical examination

GENERAL EXAMINATION
Marked cyanosis and clubbing (venous blood in aorta).

JUGULAR VENOUS PRESSURE
Giant *a* wave (right atrial hypertrophy from obstruction to outflow).

CARDIAC IMPULSES
Left ventricular hypertrophy (small right ventricle with left ventricle sustaining both circulations).

AUSCULTATION
Single second sound (P_2 absent due to low pulmonary arterial pressure). Murmurs of whichever communication is present (pansystolic murmur of ventricular septal defect or continuous murmur of persistent ductus).

Electrocardiogram
Left axis deviation is the characteristic feature, often with a P pulmonale (right atrial hypertrophy) and left ventricular hypertrophy.

Chest X-ray
The right atrium and left ventricle are large, but the pulmonary artery is small with ischaemic lung fields (except in type IIb).

Cardiac catheterization and angiography
The catheter cannot be passed into the right ventricle, but easily enters left atrium and ventricle, where the oxygen saturation is low. Angiography delineates the type of tricuspid atresia.

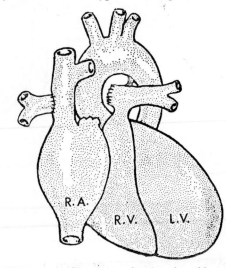

FIG. 12.17   Glenn operation for tricuspid atresia

Prognosis

Few survive infancy.

Treatment

Treatment is necessarily palliative. Aorto-pulmonary shunt operations (Blalock or Waterston) cause an increased load on an already overloaded left ventricle and are not indicated in infancy, unless the infant is very cyanosed.

Glenn operation (Fig. 12.17)
Anastomosis of the superior vena cava to the right pulmonary artery allows systemic venous blood to enter the lungs without passing through the left ventricle.

EBSTEIN'S ANOMALY

Anatomy

Abnormal position of the tricuspid valve. The posterior leaflet of the tricuspid valve is attached near the apex of the right ventricle rather than to the annulus fibrosus. The part of the ventricle above the valve is thin walled and dilated, the atrium proper is dilated and there is usually an atrial septal defect (Fig. 12.18).

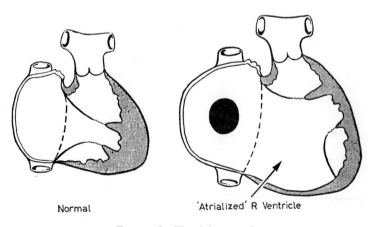

Normal   'Atrialized' R Ventricle

FIG. 12.18   Ebstein's anomaly

Haemodynamics

The tricuspid valve is incompetent and the right ventricle abnormal, with part of it contracting in continuity with the right atrium. Both factors tend to cause a low pulmonary blood flow with a high right atrial pressure.

When there is a large atrial septal defect, the right atrium decompresses itself by shunting blood into the left atrium. These patients are cyanosed and have lower right atrial pressures than those without an atrial septal defect.

Arrhythmias are common due to associated Wolff-Parkinson-White syndrome in 20% (p. 89).

Clinical Presentation

Wide spectrum of presentation. From cyanotic infant with large heart and cardiac failure, through late presentation with arrhythmias to normal life span with small heart.

Symptoms

Fatigue and dyspnoea (low cardiac output and right to left shunt). Palpitations (arrhythmias) are common.

Clinical Examination

GENERAL APPEARANCE
Cyanosis and clubbing (patients with an atrial septal defect and right to left shunt) or no cyanosis (no septal defect). The incidence of cyanosis increases with age.

J.V.P.
Normal or only slightly raised in cyanotic patients (atrium decompressed by atrial septal defect), high with a systolic wave in acyanotic patients (tricuspid regurgitation and part of RV contracting in right atrium).

CARDIAC IMPULSES
No right nor left ventricular hypertrophy.

AUSCULTATION
Clicks (late, asynchronous closure of tricuspid valve). Unusual murmurs at the lower left sternal edge in systole and diastole, sounding superficial and scratching in quality (blood flowing to and fro across the abnormal tricuspid valve). Wide split of second sound

(delayed P_2 from right bundle branch block and prolonged contraction of abnormal right ventricle).

ECG
Large P waves (right atrial hypertrophy).
Twenty per cent have Wolff-Parkinson-White syndrome. QRS complexes show a bizarre right bundle branch block pattern in 80%.

Chest X-ray
A globular *pear shaped* heart is characteristic (large right atrium and right ventricle) with abnormally clear lung fields (poor pulmonary blood flow).

Cardiac catheterization and angiography
Necessary to exclude other operable lesions such as severe pulmonary valve stenosis with a right to left shunt at atrial level. Arrhythmias during catheterization can be dangerous.

The pulmonary artery and right ventricular systolic pressures are normal. Pressure in the right atrium is high if there is no atrial septal defect, and a right atrial pressure is still obtained when the position of the catheter appears to be in the right ventricle which is confirmed with an intracavitary ECG. Angiography shows displacement of the tricuspid valve into the right ventricle.

Prognosis

Deaths from arrhythmias are common.

Treatment

Prosthetic replacement of the tricuspid valve is performed for severely disabled cases. The necessity for obliteration of the *atrialized* portion of the ventricle is debated.

TOTAL ANOMALOUS PULMONARY VENOUS DRAINAGE

Embryology

If the normal pulmonary venous outgrowth from the sinus venosus fails completely to connect with the lung, the pulmonary veins will join the venous system at some other point, either above the heart (left or right innominate veins), at heart level (coronary sinus or right

I

atrium) or below the heart (inferior vena cava, hepatic or portal veins etc.). An atrial septal defect is necessary for survival to allow the common venous return to the right atrium to reach the left atrium.

Types

Describes site of junction of common pulmonary vein with the heart:
1   *Type I*—Left innominate vein and superior vena cava (60% of cases, Fig. 12.19*a*).
2   *Type II*—Coronary sinus or right atrium (30% of cases, Fig. 12.19*b*).
3   *Type III*—Portal system.
4   *Type IV*—Multiple sites of entry.

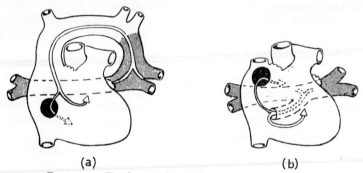

(a)   (b)

FIG. 12.19   Total anomalous pulmonary venous drainage

Haemodynamics

Pulmonary venous blood mixes with caval blood in the right atrium and flows to both ventricles, reaching the left side of the heart through an atrial communication. All chambers of the heart therefore contain blood at the same oxygen saturation.

The larger part of the venous return flows through the right ventricle and pulmonary artery because of the lower resistance to filling of the right side of the heart. The fully saturated pulmonary venous component is therefore much larger than the systemic venous component in the right atrial blood. Cyanosis is minimal, becoming marked only when the pulmonary vascular resistance rises.

Clinical Presentation

Presents like an atrial septal defect but with slight cyanosis and a *cottage loaf* chest X-ray (Type I) or severe cyanosis, oedematous lungs and early death (Type III).

Clinical examination

GENERAL
Underweight infant with slight cyanosis.

J.V.P.
Normal.

CARDIAC IMPULSES
Right ventricular hypertrophy (large left to right shunt accommodated by right heart).

AUSCULTATION
As in atrial septal defect (p. 195).

ECG
Right axis deviation and right ventricular hypertrophy (volume overload of right ventricle).

Chest X-ray
All types have large right atrium, ventricle and pulmonary artery with pulmonary plethora. In addition, Type I has a *cottage loaf* or *figure of 8* deformity consisting of the enlarged heart and the anomalous veins above it (left ascending vein joining large innominate vein and superior vena cava).

Cardiac catheterization and angiocardiography
A rise in oxygen saturation is detected at the site of entrance of the common pulmonary vein. The oxygen saturations in all chambers of the heart are similar. The exact anatomy of the pulmonary veins can be shown by angiography.

Prognosis
Most infants (80%) die during the first year.

Treatment

1   *Type I*—Using cardiopulmonary bypass with or without profound hypothermia the common pulmonary vein is anastomosed to the left atrium, the left innominate connection is ligated, and the atrial septal defect is closed.
2   *Type II*—The coronary sinus is slit to open it into the left atrium, and the atrial septal defect is closed.

DEXTROCARDIA

Definition

The heart and its apex are directed to the right.

Types

True dextrocardia as part of situs inversus (Fig. 12.20)
All viscera are transposed making a mirror image of the normal. The cavae and right atrium are to the left of the midline while the bulk of the heart is on the right. It is usually otherwise normal. The stomach and liver are transposed. A syndrome of true dextrocardia, bronchiectasis and abnormal paranasal sinuses is termed Kartagener's syndrome.

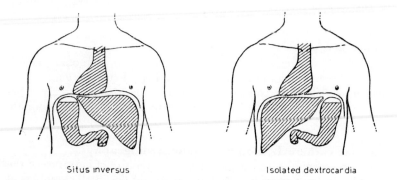

Situs inversus   Isolated dextrocardia

FIG. 12.20   Types of dextrocardia

Isolated dextrocardia (Fig. 12.20)
The viscera are in the normal position and the heart has rotated or swung round to the right so that the main bulk of the heart lies to the right of the midline. In contra-distinction to true dextrocardia with situs inversus, the cavae and right atrium are on the right. Congenital malformations of the heart are common, particularly a single ventricle.

LAEVOCARDIA

A normally placed heart in association with inversion of the abdominal viscera (Fig. 12.21). The heart is usually grossly abnormal.

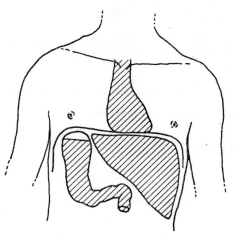

FIG. 12.21   Laevocardia

COR TRIATRIATUM

Definition

A membrane with a perforation in it divides the left atrium into two. The membrane usually separates the pulmonary veins from the mitral valve.

Clinical Presentation

The symptoms and signs are those of mitral stenosis (raised pulmonary venous pressure) except that on auscultation a soft continuous murmur is heard at the apex (pressure gradient across the membrane throughout the cardiac cycle).

Treatment

The membrane is divided under cardiopulmonary bypass.

ECTOPIA CORDIS

Definition

Displacement of the heart onto the outer surface of the body or into the abdominal cavity.

Types

1 Cervical.
2 Thoracic (the heart comes through a sternal defect).
3 Abdominal (the heart lies in the abdominal cavity or comes through a defect in the abdominal wall).
4 Thoraco-abdominal.

Prognosis

Survival for many years is possible if the heart is covered with pericardium and skin.

CHAPTER 13
DISEASES OF THE THORACIC AORTA

ANOMALIES OF THE AORTIC ARCH

Embryology

The six branchial arches each have an artery connecting ventral to dorsal aorta on either side of the foregut (trachea and oesophagus) (Fig. 13.1*a*). The first, second and fifth arches disappear. The third arch forms the carotid arteries, the fourth arch the aortic arch and right subclavian artery, and the sixth arch the pulmonary arteries and ductus arteriosus (Fig. 13.1*b*).

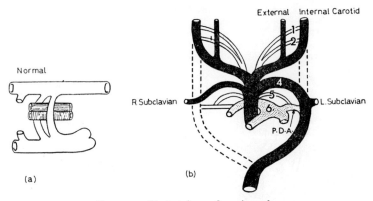

FIG. 13.1   Embryology of aortic arch

Anomalies Causing Obstruction to Trachea and Oesophagus

All the following anomalies may exist without causing obstruction. Obstruction occurs when a tight ring is formed around the trachea and oesophagus, or when an anomalous artery kinks the lumen of either.

Right aortic arch (Fig. 13.2*a*)
A right aortic arch alone causes no obstruction, but forms a ring when associated with a left ductus passing behind the oesophagus to the right arch.

Double aortic arch (Fig. 13.2*b*)
Both arches persist, one usually smaller than the other.

Aberrant subclavian artery (Fig. 13.2*c*)
A right subclavian artery arising from a left arch (or left from a right arch) passes behind the oesophagus and may kink it.

Aberrant innominate and carotid arteries (Fig. 13.2*d*)
An innominate artery arising on the left, or left common carotid on the right, may kink the trachea as it crosses it.

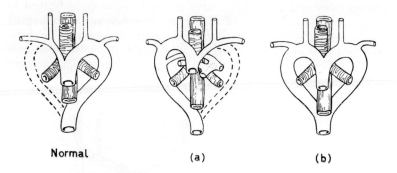

Normal   (a)   (b)

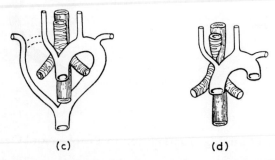

(c)   (d)

FIG. 13.2   Aortic arch anomalies causing obstruction. (a) Right sided aorta (with L. ductus behind oesophagus to R. arch). (b) Double aortic arch. (c) Anomalous R. subclavian artery. (d) Anomalous innominate or carotid arteries (after Grant)

Clinical Presentation

Only a small proportion have symptoms, which usually present in infancy.

Tracheal obstruction

Wheezing, cough, stridor, pneumonia: obstruction seen on broncho-scopy.

Oesophageal obstruction

Dysphagia (*lusoria*): obstruction seen on opaque swallow. Confirma-tion of diagnosis by simultaneous aortogram and barium swallow.

Treatment

1 Right aortic arch with left ductus—divide ductus.
2 Double aortic arch—divide smaller arch.
3 Aberrant subclavian artery—divide at origin.
4 Aberrant innominate artery—free and fix to sternum.

The fascia accompanying an artery is divided with it, as obstruction may otherwise persist after operation.

COARCTATION OF THE AORTA

Definition

Coarctation is a congenital narrowing of the aorta. In 98% of cases the coarctation is immediately distal to the origin of the left sub-clavian artery.

Types

Nomenclature is difficult as no recognized name embodies the essential difference between the two types, a difference which is physiological rather than anatomical.

Descending aorta supplied from the aortic arch (*post-ductal, adult*)

Blood reaches the lower half of the body through the coarctation and collateral vessels. If a persistent ductus arteriosus is present, blood flows from aorta to pulmonary artery regardless of the position of the ductus in relation to the coarctation. This type may present at any time from infancy to old age.

Descending aorta supplied from the pulmonary artery (*preductal, infantile*)

The distal aorta below the coarctation is really a continuation of the ductus arteriosus and the lower body receives pulmonary venous blood from the pulmonary artery, mixed with some arterial blood

flowing through the coarctation. This type usually presents in
infancy because it is often associated with other congenital cardiac
anomalies such as a ventricular septal defect which maintains a high
pressure and oxygen saturation in the pulmonary artery, ductus and
lower limbs. There is little stimulus to the formation of collateral
vessels.

Haemodynamics of the Adult Type (Fig. 13.3)

The constriction in the aorta results in the following:

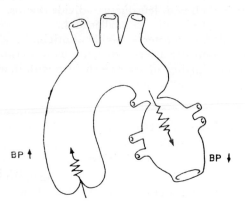

FIG. 13.3   Haemodynamics of coarctation

Proximal hypertension
The blood pressure in the head and arms above the coarctation is
elevated for reasons that are not clear, neither the mechanical
obstruction to blood flow nor the effects of a small pulse pressure on
the kidneys adequately explaining the hypertension.

Hypertension gives the left ventricle an extra work load and the
increased cerebral arterial pressure predisposes to cerebral haemorrhage. Very high pressures occur during exertion.

Turbulence at the narrowed segment
Blood forced through the narrowed orifice causes turbulence—the
coarctation murmur.

Distal hypotension and delayed femoral pulses
The blood flow to the body beyond the coarctation is maintained by
collateral vessels which arise above the coarctation from branches of
the subclavian artery and empty into the aorta below the coarctation. Anteriorly the internal mammary artery communicates with

the anterior intercostal arteries, laterally axillary artery branches communicate with the lateral cutaneous branches of the intercostal arteries, and posteriorly the superior intercostal artery communicates with posterior intercostal branches.

These collateral vessels are large and numerous so that the mean blood pressure distally is often normal but the pulse pressure is reduced and there is a delay in the transmission of the pulse wave to the aorta beyond the coarctation. The first few pairs of aortic intercostal arteries carry the largest flow of blood, which makes them tortuous and they erode the under surface of the ribs.

Commonly associated abnormalities are a bicuspid aortic valve (common cause of aortic ejection murmur)—small congenital aneurysms on the cerebral arteries—aortic stenosis and regurgitation—persistent ductus arteriosus—*left heart syndrome* (hypoplasia of the left heart, congenital mitral stenosis, endocardial fibro-elastosis, aortic stenosis and coarctation of the aorta)—anomalous origin of subclavian arteries. Either the right or the left subclavian artery may arise below the coarctation.

Clinical Presentation of Post-ductal, Adult Type

Usually presents as a chance finding of hypertension in the arms with a diminished and delayed femoral pulse.

Symptoms
1   Usually none (60%). The diagnosis is made at a routine medical examination.
2   Proximal hypertension may cause dyspnoea on exertion and finally frank left ventricular failure. Cerebral arterial hypertension and cerebral aneurysms may result in cerebro-vascular accidents.
3   Turbulence at an associated bicuspid aortic valve or at the narrowed segment predisposes to subacute bacterial endarteritis.
4   Intermittent claudication and cold feet are not prominent symptoms for blood flow is usually good below the coarctation.

Clinical examination

GENERAL
Disproportionate build with well developed shoulders and thin legs (collateral vessels in shoulder muscles).

PULSES AND BLOOD PRESSURE
1   Brachial, suprasternal and carotid pulsation are of increased amplitude and the blood pressure in the arms is raised.

2   The femoral pulses are small (small pulse pressure) and delayed compared with the radial pulses (effect of constriction in the aorta and long course of pulse wave via collateral vessels).

3   Palpable collateral arteries are felt around the scapulae, best appreciated with the patient leaning forward and the arms crossed across the chest.

CARDIAC IMPULSES
Forceful apical impulse (left ventricular hypertrophy).

AUSCULTATION
Aortic ejection click and ejection murmur in 60% (associated bicuspid aortic valve). A systolic murmur is heard at the back to the left of the vertebral column at the 4th intercostal space (turbulence at the coarctation). It is distinguished from the systolic murmur produced by collateral vessels in the back muscles by becoming louder instead of being obliterated by heavy pressure with the stethoscope.

Electrocardiography
Left ventricular hypertrophy.

Chest X-ray
1   Abnormal aortic knuckle. Characteristically the dilated left subclavian artery is visible as a prominent bulge above the coarctation with poststenotic dilatation of the aorta below.

2   Rib notching (collateral blood flow along the aortic intercostal arteries makes them tortuous and erodes the under border of the ribs). Maximal in the intercostal spaces of the first intercostal arteries arising from the aorta (3rd, 4th and 5th).

3   Little enlargement of the cardiac shadow (left ventricular hypertrophy rather than dilatation).

Cardiac catheterization and angiography
Not normally indicated because the site and the severity of the coarctation is obvious on clinical grounds.

1   The diagnosis of a narrowed area of aorta beyond the left subclavian artery is made by delay of the femoral pulse compared with the radial.

2   The severity of the coarctation is indicated by the degree of diminution and delay of the femoral pulse, the presence of collateral vessels and the height of the blood pressure in the arms.

3   The site of the coarctation is shown by the position of the coarctation murmur in the back and by those ribs showing maximal notching being the ones immediately distal to the narrowing.

Retrograde femoral aortic catheterization, for measurement of the pressure gradient across the coarctation and angiography, is indicated only when the coarctation is atypical (i.e. minimal diminution and delay of the femoral pulse, suspected abnormal site of the coarctation or anomalous subclavian arteries).

Other Types of Coarctation

'Preductal', 'infantile' coarctation

PRESENTATION
This type of coarctation is commonly associated with other congenital anomalies, long atretic segments of the aorta and poor development of collateral vessels. It presents usually with heart failure in infancy, although some patients survive to older childhood.

DIFFERENTIAL DIAGNOSIS FROM 'POSTDUCTAL' 'ADULT' TYPE
1 The feet may be bluer than the hands, though this sign is rarely marked because there is almost invariably a ventricular septal defect which raises the oxygen content of the blood flowing into the pulmonary artery.
2 Angiography will demonstrate the anatomy.

Abdominal and lower thoracic coarctation
Two per cent of all coarctations. The coarctation murmur is low in the thorax or abdomen and on the chest X-ray the aortic knuckle is normal and rib notching affects the lower ribs only.

Anomalous subclavian arteries
A diminished and delayed pulse in one arm compared with the other indicates a subclavian artery arising below the coarctation. Angiography is necessary for confirmation.

Prognosis

Ninety per cent of patients with coarctation die before the age of 40, most commonly from cardiac failure in infancy.

If infancy is survived, the average life expectancy is 33 years, death due to coarctation being caused by:
1 Rupture of the aorta (dissecting aneurysms of proximal aorta) in one third.
2 Subacute bacterial endarteritis (usually on a bicuspid aortic valve) in one third.

3   Effects of systemic hypertension (left ventricular failure and cerebral haemorrhage) in one third.

Surgical Treatment

Indications
All typical coarctations are recommended for surgery on diagnosis because of their poor prognosis. The optimal age for operation is 7–15.

Exceptions
1   Mild coarctations (normal blood pressure and no femoral arterial delay).
2   Infancy, unless cardiac failure is unresponsive to medical treatment.

The operative mortality and recurrence rate is high in infancy but the risks are justifiable in the few who do not respond to medical treatment.

Technique (Fig. 13.4)
The aorta is occluded, the coarctation resected and an end to end anastomosis performed. If the gap is too large, a crimped woven Dacron graft is inserted to establish continuity or a lateral patch used after excising the shelf of the coarctation itself.

Results
Symptoms are relieved and blood pressure reduced, though not always to normal. The incidence of surgical complications varies with the age of the patient:
1   *Infancy.*
　　(i)   Operative mortality 70% under 3 months.
　　(ii) Recurrence of coarctation 25%.
2   *After infancy.*
　　(i)   Mortality 2–6% (haemorrhage and infection of the anastomosis).
　　(ii) Morbidity (hypertensive crises of unknown aetiology, mesenteric arteritis due to the unaccustomed pulse pressure, recurrent nerve palsy).
3   *Over 40 years of age.*
Operative mortality 12% but relief of symptoms and reduction of blood pressure is comparable to those under 40 years of age.

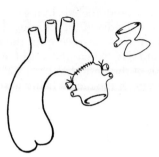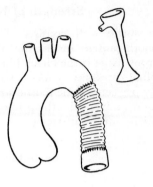

END TO END ANASTOMOSIS   **GRAFT**

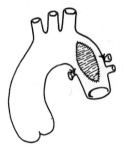

PATCH

FIG. 13.4   Operations for coarctation of the aorta

ANEURYSMS OF THE THORACIC AORTA

Definition

An aortic aneurysm is a localized dilatation of the aortic wall. Aneurysms may be subdivided for descriptive purposes into saccular, fusiform and dissecting types, although dissections are not localized and strictly do not fit the definition of an aneurysm.

Strength of Normal Aortic Wall

The aortic wall consists of intima (endothelial lining), media (smooth muscle and elastic tissue) and adventitia (fibrous tissue). Fibrous tissue is the check fibre which resists stretch until the intraluminal pressure reaches 1000 mm Hg when the aorta bursts. Sixty per cent of the tensile strength of the aorta has been shown to lie in the adventitia, the prime function of the media being to supply elasticity, and not strength.

Pathology of Aneurysms

Saccular and fusiform aneurysms

SYPHILITIC

The proximal aorta is affected most frequently. Round cell infiltration and endarteritis are accompanied by necrosis and fibrous tissue replacement. The healed syphilitic aorta is entirely replaced with fibrous tissue and can be shown, as expected from the above, to be many times stronger than the normal aorta. Saccular aneurysms begin at the inflammatory stage if necrosis outstrips fibrous tissue replacement in localized areas.

ARTERIOSCLEROTIC

Intimal atheromatous plaques involve the media and adventitia secondarily, weakening the aorta and producing fusiform aneurysms usually of the descending aorta.

TRAUMATIC (Fig. 13.5)

The thoracic aorta is fixed to other structures at its origin, at the site of the ligamentum arteriosum, and at the diaphragm. Sudden deceleration, as in a car crash, may tear the aorta at these points when the remainder of the aorta is carried forward by the momentum of its contained blood. The aorta tears most often above the aortic valve in the pericardium when death is usually instantaneous from tamponade. Less commonly it tears at the ligamentum, and 10–20% of these patients survive with the blood contained by surrounding fibrous tissue to form an aneurysm.

OTHER CAUSES

Congenital, mycotic, cystic medionecrosis. The last may produce a markedly dilated ascending aorta and aortic regurgitation ('triple sinus aneurysm', 'aortic annulo-ectasia') with or without a dissection.

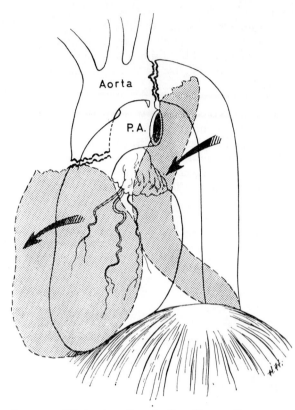

FIG. 13.5 Mechanism of production of traumatic aneurysms

Dissecting aneurysms

DEFINITION
The entry and spread of blood into and along the media.

AETIOLOGY
Only an abnormal aortic media can be dissected in this way. A physical change in the media allows its layers to separate easily, a change usually associated with cystic medial necrosis in which muco-polysaccharide is laid down between degenerating elastic fibres. The aetiology of cystic medial necrosis is not known but it occurs in association with Marfan's syndrome (arachnodactyly, dislocation of the lenses, high arched palate, pigeon chest and muscular hypotonia), coarctation, pregnancy and lathyrism (ingestion of sweet pea oil). Dissections are often associated with systemic hypertension.

PATHOLOGY

An intimal tear allows blood to enter the media and spread along it, flattening the true lumen, occluding large branches of the aorta and shearing off small ones. The intimal tear may be initiated by a haemorrhage in the media, by an atheromatous plaque or occur spontaneously.

TYPES OF DISSECTING ANEURYSM (Figs. 13.6 and 13.11)

Type I   The most common type, beginning in the ascending aorta and spreading round to the descending.

Type II   Aneurysm confined to the ascending aorta.

Type III   Dissection begins in the descending aorta and may be confined to it or extend into the abdominal aorta.

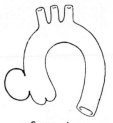

Saccular

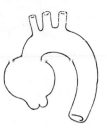

Fusiform

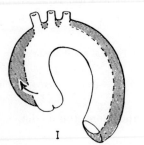

I

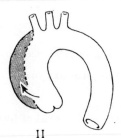

II

Dissecting

FIG. 13.6   Ascending aorta. Surgical problems

Clinical Presentation

Saccular and fusiform aneurysms

SYMPTOMS

1   Often asymptomatic (chance finding on X-ray).

2   Pressure effects on neighbouring structures:
   (i) Bronchus (pneumonia, wheeze).
   (ii) Oesophagus (dysphagia).
   (iii) Sternum and vertebrae (pain).
   (iv) Recurrent laryngeal nerve (hoarseness).

CLINICAL EXAMINATION
Usually no abnormal signs. Depending on the site of the aneurysm
there may be visible pulsation (ascending aorta), tracheal tug (arch
pushing down left main bronchus at each pulse beat), and *cogwheel*
breathing (compression of bronchus with each pulse beat).

CHEST X-RAY
1   Mass associated with aorta on postero-anterior and lateral
views.
2   Tomography may show calcification of aneurysmal wall.

ANGIOGRAPHY
1   Information required:
   (i) Confirmation that mass is an aortic aneurysm.
   (ii) Number of involved aortic branches.
   (iii) Contained clot (disparity in size of aneurysmal lumen compared with its external dimensions).
   (iv) Width of neck of sac.
2   Route.
Injection in the aorta gives the best contrast but may cause the
aneurysm to rupture or dislodge thrombus. Injection in the right
heart is safe but gives poorer contrast.

Dissecting aneurysms

SYMPTOMS
1   Severe tearing pain in chest (ascending aortic dissection), back
(descending) or abdomen (abdominal dissection).
2   Symptoms of infarction of organs supplied by blocked aortic
branches (cerebral, spinal, renal or mesenteric arterial occlusion can
give a wide variety of symptoms).

CLINICAL EXAMINATION
1   Shocked patient in severe pain.
2   Aortic regurgitation (if dissection has detached an aortic cusp).
3   Murmurs in back or abdomen (occluded lumen).
4   Absent pulses in branches involved by the dissection.

ELECTROCARDIOGRAPHY

No typical feature. May show left ventricular hypertrophy (previous systemic hypertension). Evidence of myocardial ischaemia does not exclude dissection because an infarct may have occurred in the past or the dissection may be occluding a coronary artery.

CHEST X-RAY

A wide mediastinum suggests the diagnosis. Increasing width on serial radiographs is diagnostic.

ANGIOGRAPHY

Information required before treatment can be planned:

1 Confirmation of diagnosis (twin lumen of false and true channels).
2 Extent of aneurysm and branches involved.
3 Site of intimal tear.

Prognosis

Saccular and fusiform aneurysms

LIFE EXPECTANCY

Fifty per cent die within 5 years, 70% within 10 years (comparable figures for patients of same age groups without aneurysms 10% and 20%).

CAUSES OF DEATH

1 Rupture.
2 Pressure on surrounding structures (common with syphilitic aneurysms, rare in arteriosclerotic ones).
3 Cardiac failure (from aortic regurgitation in syphilitic aneurysms and from associated coronary disease in arteriosclerotic cases).
4 Arteriosclerosis elsewhere (particularly of the cerebral vessels).

FACTORS CARRYING A POOR PROGNOSIS

1 Large aneurysm.
2 Aneurysm causing symptoms.
The interval between the onset of symptoms and death in untreated syphilitic aneurysms is 10–20 months.
3 Age over 50.
4 Systemic hypertension.
5 Arteriosclerosis elsewhere (cerebral, coronary, abdominal aorta).

Dissecting aneurysms

LIFE EXPECTANCY

One-fifth die in 24 hours, half in four days, nine-tenths in three months. Five year survival 1%.

CAUSES OF DEATH

1 Acute (within 2 weeks) —almost all due to rupture.
2 Subacute (2–6 weeks)—most due to rupture but a quarter die of late effects of ischaemia from occluded branches.
3 Chronic (after 6 weeks)—majority due to rupture but one-third from cardiac failure (aortic regurgitation).

Treatment

Indications for surgery

SACCULAR AND FUSIFORM ANEURYSMS

1 Large or enlarging aneurysm.
2 Symptoms from the aneurysm.
3 Embolism.

DISSECTING ANEURYSMS

Treatment of acute dissecting aneurysms is conservative, lowering the blood pressure and reducing the rate of rise of pressure in the aorta with beta blocking agents. If there is evidence of blockage of important arteries or severe aortic regurgitation in the acute phase, or if there is continued enlargement or extension in the chronic phase, surgery is recommended.

Technique

ASCENDING AORTIC ANEURYSM (Figs. 13.7 and 13.8)

Cardiopulmonary bypass with coronary artery perfusion.
1 Saccular aneurysm. Excised and the neck sutured directly if it is narrow, or patched with Dacron if it is more than one third of the circumference of the aorta.
2 Fusiform aneurysm. Excised and the ascending aorta replaced with a Dacron graft (Fig. 13.7). Triple sinus aneurysms require aortic valve replacement with, if necessary, transplantation of the coronary arteries to the graft (Fig. 13.7).
3 Type I dissecting aneurysms (extending beyond the ascending aorta). The aorta is divided at the level of the intimal tear, oversewing the double lumen distally and re-anastomosing the aorta. Blood is thus directed into the true lumen (Fig. 13.8).

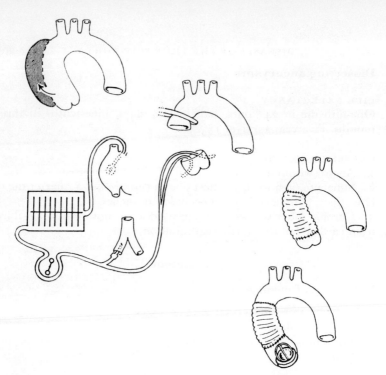

FIG. 13.7 Ascending aorta. Surgery of Type II dissecting aneurysm (illustrated) or fusiform aneurysm

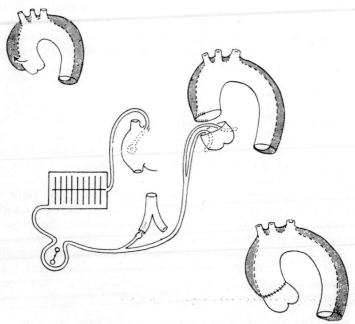

FIG. 13.8 Ascending aorta. Surgery of Type I dissecting aneurysm

4 Type II dissecting aneurysms (confined to the ascending aorta). The ascending aorta is replaced with a graft. Aortic regurgitation is particularly common in this type and the aortic valve may have to be replaced also (Fig. 13.7).

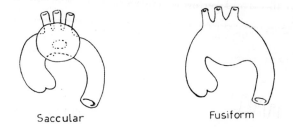

Saccular   Fusiform

Fig. 13.9 Aortic arch. Surgical problems

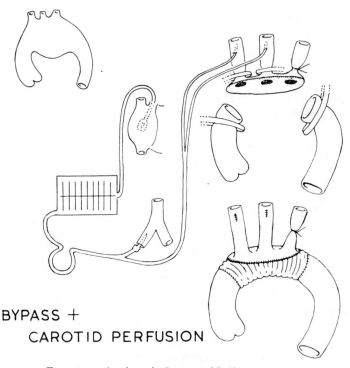

BYPASS +
CAROTID PERFUSION

Fig. 13.10 Aortic arch. Surgery of fusiform aneurysm

AORTIC ARCH (Fig. 13.9)

1 Saccular aneurysms are best treated by lateral aortorrhaphy—placing a clamp across the neck and excising it except for a cuff which is oversewn—or the neck is sutured directly using profound hypothermia and circulatory arrest.

Saccular aneurysms with a wide neck require cardiopulmonary bypass with carotid perfusion while the sac is excised and the aorta patched.

Fusiform aneurysms are treated by excision and graft replacement (Fig. 13.10).

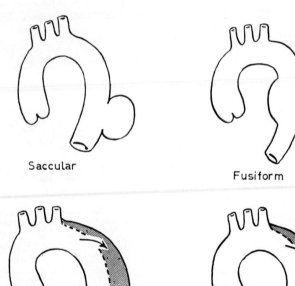

Saccular   Fusiform

Dissecting III

Fig. 13.11   Descending aorta. Surgical problems

DESCENDING THORACIC AORTA (Fig. 13.11)

A bypass around the occluded descending aorta is used, from left atrium through a pump to the femoral artery (Fig. 13.12).

1 Saccular aneurysms. Excised and patched.
2 Fusiform aneurysms. Excised and replaced with a Dacron graft.

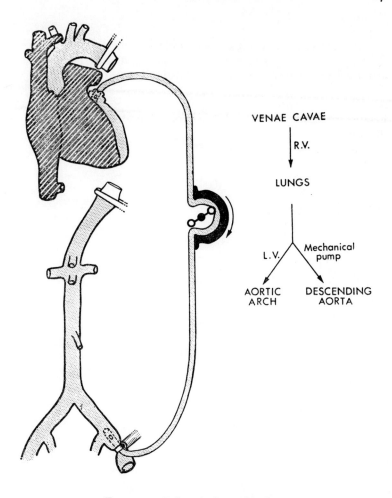

VENAE CAVAE

R.V.

LUNGS

L.V.   Mechanical
        pump

AORTIC   DESCENDING
ARCH   AORTA

Fig. 13.12   Left atrio-femoral bypass

3   Type III dissecting aneurysms confined to the thorax are totally excised and replaced with a graft.

4   Type III dissecting aneurysms extending into the abdomen. The double lumen is oversewn distally before anastomosing the graft, directing blood back into the true lumen.

Results

SACCULAR AND FUSIFORM ANEURYSMS

Factors increasing mortality: old age, systemic hypertension, arteriosclerosis elsewhere, and pre-existing heart disease.

DISSECTING ANEURYSMS

Factors increasing mortality: systemic hypertension and cardiac disease.

CHAPTER 14
ISCHAEMIC HEART DISEASE

Ischaemic heart disease is the leading cause of death in all affluent countries. There are over 138,000 deaths in the United Kingdom each year caused by ischaemic heart disease and more than half of the men are under 65 when they die.

Definition

The coronary blood flow is insufficient for the needs of the heart owing to disease of the coronary arteries.

Aetiology

Atheroma of the coronary arteries
This is by far the most frequent cause of ischaemic heart disease. Syphilitic coronary ostial stenosis, polyarteritis nodosa and coronary artery embolism are rare lesions also causing narrowing or obstruction of the coronary arteries.

PATHOLOGY
Atheroma is a degenerative disease, involving the deposition of plaques of lipoid material in the intima of the coronary arteries. These plaques are almost always multiple, compromising or occluding the lumen of the main coronary arteries and their larger branches. Thrombus formation on a plaque may further narrow or occlude the artery.

CAUSE OF CORONARY ATHEROMA
Atheroma is a local manifestation in the arterial wall of a general disturbance of lipid transport. The identified 'risk factors' for the subsequent development of clinical ischaemic heart disease are male sex, increasing age, raised levels of the systemic blood pressure, raised blood cholesterol and cigarette smoking. A high risk man has a one in three chance of developing clinical ischaemic heart disease within a ten year period.

Male sex
Ischaemic heart disease is six times more frequent in men than

women aged 40–50, but this difference steadily declines with increasing age.

Age

The numbers of hospital admissions rise to a peak in middle aged men. The numbers of cases decline in the older age groups only because the size of the population at risk diminishes. The incidence and mortality rates rise throughout life, approximately doubling for every 10 years of advancing age.

Blood pressure

The incidence of ischaemic heart disease and cerebrovascular disease rises with increasing levels of the systemic blood pressure. Reduction of the blood pressure has considerable effect in the prevention of cerebrovascular disease but little, if any, on ischaemic heart disease.

Cholesterol

A serum cholesterol of over 225 mg % carries with it an increased risk of ischaemic heart disease.

Disturbances of fat metabolism, many having a high incidence of ischaemic heart disease, are classified from the lipoprotein pattern of the fasting serum. These hyperlipoproteinaemias may be familial or secondary to hypothyroidism, diabetes mellitus, the nephrotic syndrome and biliary obstruction.

The Hyperlipoproteinaemias

Type	Lipoprotein abnormality	Lipid abnormality	Treatment
I	Chylomicra present	Triglycerides +++	Restrict fat in diet
IIa	Beta lipoprotein raised	Cholesterol ++	Cholestyramine or clofibrate
IIb	Beta and prebeta raised	Cholesterol + Triglycerides +	Low fat, low carbohydrate diet ± clofibrate
III	Broad beta present	Cholesterol ++ Triglycerides ++	as above
IV	Prebeta raised	Triglycerides ++	Reduce carbohydrate intake
V	Chylomicra present prebeta raised	Triglycerides +++ Cholesterol +	Diet and clofibrate

Cigarette smoking

The risk of ischaemic heart disease is increased several fold in men up to the age of 55, and the risk of sudden death is especially increased. When smoking is given up, the excess risk is gradually lost after 5–10 years.

Other probable risk factors
Faulty diet, obesity, physical inactivity, emotional stress, hardness of water supply, glucose in tolerance, high serum uric acid and family history of coronary artery disease.

CLINICAL SYNDROMES OF ISCHAEMIC HEART DISEASE

Narrowing of the coronary arteries presents with the clinical syndromes of angina pectoris, acute coronary insufficiency, and myocardial infarction. Cardiac failure, sudden death or cardiac arrhythmias may also be presenting features.

Angina Pectoris

Description
Angina pectoris occurs when the blood supply to the myocardium is temporarily insufficient; lactic acid and other metabolites accumulate in the anoxic myocardium, stimulate nerve endings and cause pain.

Symptoms
Chest pain is the principal symptom and the diagnosis of angina pectoris is made from the characteristic features of this pain:
Site and radiation The pain is retrosternal or spreads across the front of the chest. It may radiate into the angle of the jaws, through to the back and down both arms into the fingers.
Character Tight, band like, heavy or crushing, but not sharp.
Relation to exercise Comes on during physical exertion forcing the patient to stop, when it eases off within three to five minutes. The pain does not last for only seconds nor does it continue for 20 minutes. Walking uphill after breakfast is the most common single time for angina to occur, especially if it is uphill against a cold wind. Some patients can continue walking until the angina subsides but this attempt at a 'second wind' in angina is dangerous. Mental excitement or anger may precipitate an attack.

Variants of angina pectoris
Angina decubitus Pain on lying flat relieved by sitting up.

Implies involvement of all three main coronary arteries and is accompanied by severe angina of effort.

Nocturnal angina Patient wakens from sleep with angina, possibly provoked by vivid dreams.

Prinzmetal's angina A rare form where pain comes on without relation to exercise, the electrocardiogram showing ST elevation during the pain. Many progress to myocardial infarction.

Clinical examination

Physical examination will exclude other causes of angina pectoris not directly attributable to coronary artery disease—aortic stenosis, anaemia, cardiac arrhythmias, severe pulmonary hypertension. In the large majority of patients in whom angina pectoris is the result of coronary atheroma there is no abnormality on clinical examination. Occasionally evidence of a condition favouring atheroma is found, such as systemic hypertension or a manifestation of a hyperlipidaemia:

1 Tendon xanthomas indicate a hyperbetalipoproteinaemia of Type II.

2 Planar xanthomas on the palms of the hands occur in Type III and in homozygotes for Type II.

3 Xanthelasma (yellow plaques in the eyelids) is frequent in Type II and occasionally occurs in Type III but is often seen in the absence of any hyperlipidaemia.

4 Arcus senilis (narrow grey line of cholesterol deposit in the margin of the cornea) is significant only in people below age 40. It then implies Type II hyperlipoproteinaemia.

5 Tuberous xanthomas occur in Types II and III and eruptive xanthomas in Types I and V.

Electrocardiography

ST segment depression indicating myocardial ischaemia is the characteristic feature, but the electrocardiogram is often normal at rest. The diagnosis should be made from the characteristic history alone in these patients. Where there is real doubt, an electrocardiogram during exertion will show changes in 90% of patients (there is some danger in exercising patients with ischaemic heart disease).

Chest X-ray

Normal. Calcification in the coronary arteries on fluoroscopy indicates coronary atheroma but is no guide to the presence or degree of coronary artery obstruction.

Coronary angiography

Individual catheterization and injection of contrast into the coronary arteries show the presence and situation of obstructions.

INDICATIONS
Intractable angina when surgical treatment is under consideration.
Atypical chest pain not capable of diagnosis using all routine
methods including electrocardiography during exertion.
Aortic stenosis when coronary artery disease is a possible cause of
chest pain.

Prognosis

The average life expectancy is ten years from the onset of symptoms
but there is wide variation. Angina pectoris rapidly increasing in
severity over the course of a few days or weeks usually culminates in
myocardial infarction, whereas the frequency and severity of attacks
may remain stable for many years.

Prevention

General measures accepted as likely to delay the onset of coronary
disease in the general population are regular exercise, avoidance of
cigarette smoking and treatment of systemic hypertension. Diets low
in fat or containing a high proportion of unsaturated fatty acids
reduce the blood lipids but there is no proof that this has any effect
on atheroma formation.

Treatment

ACTIVITY
Angina occurs when myocardial work and oxygen demand exceed
the available oxygen supply. Increased heart rate and blood pressure
greatly increase the myocardial oxygen demand. Pain provoking
activities are avoided as far as possible but exercise short of producing the pain is encouraged. Moderate exertion probably stimu-
lates coronary collateral blood flow.

DIET
Low calorie diet for obese patients. A blood lipid lowering diet is not
essential as there is no good evidence that symptoms or prognosis are
improved thereby.

DRUG TREATMENT

Glyceryl trinitrate
0·5 mg tablet crushed in the teeth and dissolved in the mouth, taken
when pain begins or is anticipated. Quickly relieves pain by reducing
cardiac work rather than by acting as a coronary vasodilator. Both
cardiac output and systemic blood pressure are reduced for about 20

minutes. Headache is a side effect. Glyceryl trinitrate should be used liberally as there is no addictive effect and it does not lose efficacy with prolonged usage.

Long acting nitrites (pentaerythritol tetranitrate) and slow release glyceryl trinitrate (Sustac) are usually ineffective. For pain not controlled by glyceryl trinitrate, beta-adrenergic blocking drugs are advised.

Beta-adrenergic blocking drugs

These act in angina by slowing the heart rate, reducing the systemic blood pressure and decreasing the vigour of cardiac contraction—all giving a decrease in cardiac work. Caution is required if there is cardiac failure because all these drugs remove sympathetic drive from the heart and intensify failure. If used at all, the patient should be digitalized and the drug given in very low dosage at first.

Propranolol No intrinsic sympathetic activity. No cardiac selectivity. Dosage gradually increased to 80 mg four times daily or more. Side effects include bronchial asthma, vivid dreams and cardiac failure.

Practolol Slight intrinsic sympathetic activity. High degree of cardiac selectivity. 100 mg twice daily, gradually increasing. Bronchial asthma is less likely.

Oxprenolol High intrinsic sympathetic activity. A useful alternative to the other beta blocking drugs.

Anticoagulant therapy

Long-term anticoagulant therapy does not significantly affect the symptoms or prognosis and the risks of haemorrhage outweigh any marginal benefits.

Clofibrate

Lowers serum cholesterol, triglycerides and free fatty acids in a dosage of 1G twice daily. Quite apart from these actions it is suggested that long term therapy favourably influences the mortality of angina patients.

ADDITIONAL MEASURES IN INTRACTABLE ANGINA PECTORIS

Saphenous vein bypass graft (Fig. 14.1)

For intractable angina with a block of more than 50% of the lumen of one or more coronary arteries and a demonstrably adequate peripheral vessel. On cardiopulmonary bypass a segment of saphenous vein is anastomosed between the ascending aorta and each artery distal to the block. Mortality 4–6%. Immediate results: in 80% of patients angina is abolished or much relieved. Late results (thrombosis of grafts and effect of operation on longevity of patient): not yet known.

A variant of this operation is the direct anastomosis of the internal mammary artery to the involved coronary artery. Implantation of the internal mammary artery into a tunnel in the myocardium (Vineberg operation) has been virtually abandoned because of poor long term results.

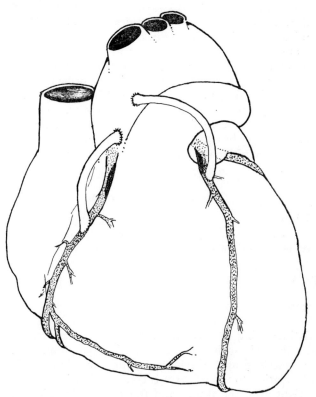

FIG. 14.1   Saphenous vein bypass graft from aorta to coronary arteries distal to a block

Acute Coronary Insufficiency

Symptoms
Symptoms of angina pectoris occur at rest with the electrocardiogram showing ST segment depression at rest. An acute change has occurred

K

in a coronary artery producing an important decrease in the lumen. Many go on to myocardial infarction but an important group persists with a blood supply just sufficient to prevent necrosis.

Prognosis
20–30% develop myocardial infarction within 3 months.

Treatment
Reduce myocardial work while heart develops a collateral circulation:
1   Bed rest for weeks with analgesics for pain and a gradual resumption of activities when pain ceases.
2   A course of anticoagulant therapy is widely used but few myocardial infarctions arise on the basis of a final thrombosis in the narrowed coronary artery and little benefit can be expected.
3   Beta blocking drugs may reduce the episodes of pain.
4   Emergency saphenous vein bypass surgery. When coronary arteriography demonstrates a readily accessible major obstruction, emergency surgery has had some success. Myocardial infarction may however be precipitated and the long term results of this surgery are not known.

Myocardial Infarction

Definition
Necrosis of an area of myocardium, almost invariably the result of gross reduction of coronary blood flow to the affected area. Fresh coronary artery platelet thrombi are found in at least half of autopsy cases.

Symptoms
1   Chest pain (over 90% of patients). Fifty per cent have had angina pectoris increasing in severity over several weeks, but in the remainder the pain of infarction is the first symptom. Pain is often intense, described as a heaviness, burning or aching in the central chest. Radiation to the left arm is common but it may also radiate to the right arm, the throat and the angles of the jaw. The pain usually persists for many hours and is not relieved by glyceryl trinitrate.
2   Less constant symptoms include dyspnoea, nausea, vomiting, perspiration and mental anguish. At the onset faintness and loss of consciousness are common, probably vasovagal in origin. Myocardial infarction may be painless, particularly in the elderly.

Clinical examination

1 Anxious patient with pallor, sweating, tachycardia or bradycardia.

2 Irregular pulse due to extrasystoles.

3 Transient systemic hypertension in first few hours, thereafter a blood pressure below usual level.

4 Jugular venous pressure slightly elevated, particularly when an inferior infarct involves the right ventricle.

5 Outward bulging of the precordium during systole—a constant finding in major anterior infarction.

6 Auscultation. Fourth heart sound (atrial gallop) almost always present. Third heart sound infrequent and indicates severe left ventricular failure. Transient pericardial friction rub on 2nd day (10%). Apical systolic murmur preceded by click—abnormal papillary muscle function (50% of patients). Sudden appearance of loud pansystolic murmur—ruptured interventricular septum (less than 0·5%) or rarely due to ruptured papillary muscle.

7 Shock. Mental confusion or apathy. Systolic blood pressure below 90 mm Hg. Pallor with cold extremities. Oliguria.

Electrocardiography

Changes are found in over 95% of patients, usually soon after the onset of pain although occasionally changes are delayed for some days (p. 48).

1 ST elevation—with onset of infarction.

2 Pathological (0·04 sec) Q waves over the infarct—within hours.

3 T inversion and return of ST segment to iso-electric line—during the next few weeks.

Persistent ST segment elevation months later indicates a left ventricular aneurysm. All the other changes can persist indefinitely or may revert to normal in the months after infarction.

Confirmatory evidence of myocardial necrosis

1 Reaction of the body to necrotic muscle:

(i) Pyrexia appearing on the second day and subsiding over the next few days.

(ii) Leucocytosis in the peripheral blood, maximal during the first few days.

(iii) Pericardial friction rub fleetingly present in the early days after infarction.

(iv) Erythrocyte sedimentation rate rising to a maximum in the second week.

2 Enzymes released into the peripheral blood by the necrotic muscle:

K*

(i) Serum glutamic oxaloacetic transaminase (SGOT, normal range 10–35 units). Increased within twelve hours, peak activity between 18–36 hours and back to normal within 3 to 4 days. Other conditions causing a raised SGOT are hepatic congestion, primary liver disease, skeletal muscle disease, shock, myocarditis, pericarditis, pulmonary embolism, tachycardia, direct current shock, ingestion of oral contraceptives or clofibrate.

(ii) Serum lactic dehydrogenase (LDH). Increased in 24 to 48 hours from onset of pain, peak activity 3–6 days, normal range after 8–14 days. Also raised in congestive heart failure, haemolytic anaemia, megaloblastic anaemia, acute and chronic liver disease, renal disease, neoplastic disease, pulmonary embolism, shock. The iso-enzyme LDH_1 is a more sensitive and more specific indicator of myocardial infarction.

(iii) Serum creatine phosphokinase (CPK). Increased within 6 to 8 hours of myocardial infarction, reaches a peak of two to tenfold in 24 hours and declines to normal within 3–4 days. Also markedly raised in muscular dystrophy, inflammatory disease of muscle, alcohol intoxication, diabetes mellitus, convulsions, psychosis and after intramuscular injections.

Prognosis
The causes of death in myocardial infarction are:
1 Primary arrhythmias (45%).
2 Pump failure, including shock (40%).
3 Cardiac rupture (10%).
4 Pulmonary or systemic embolism (3%).
5 Renal failure, infection etc. (2%).
The time of death is important. One third of all patients die within 3 hours of the onset of pain, many not reaching hospital. The coronary care unit is effective in the prevention and treatment of arrhythmias, reducing the hospital mortality from 30% to well under 20%.

The prognosis of cardiogenic shock is poor, because this indicates massive infarction—mortality over 80%.

Treatment

RAPID PAIN RELIEF
Heroin 5 mg intravenously or morphine 10 mg intravenously.

Disadvantages: further blood pressure reduction, depression of respiration, reduction of cardiac output and vomiting provoked in some patients. These drugs are not given in the absence of pain.

CONTROL OF ARRHYTHMIAS

The incidence of cardiac arrhythmia in the first hours is practically 100%.

The electrocardiogram is monitored continuously for 36 hours—the time of risk of serious arrhythmia—in a coronary care unit. Potentially serious arrhythmias are suppressed by drug therapy with immediate resuscitation available if necessary.

Ventricular extrasystoles

Very common, only the following require treatment:

1 Multifocal ventricular extrasystoles.
2 Ventricular extrasystoles close to the T wave.
3 Ventricular extrasystoles occurring more than 5 per minute.

Lignocaine 100 mg i.v. as a bolus. If this is effective a continuous infusion of lignocaine is given, 100–200 mg per hour for 36 hours. Adverse reactions are few: drowsiness, convulsions. No decrease in blood pressure or cardiac output.

Ventricular tachycardia (20% of patients)

Lignocaine 100 mg intravenously, repeated in 5 minutes if necessary, or Practolol intravenously up to a maximum of 25 mg. Sodium phenytoin may be effective in the refractory case but causes severe phlebitis in the injected vein, with nausea, vomiting, dizziness and nystagmus. Dosage 100 mg intravenously up to 600 mg.

Other measures include synchronized direct current shock used immediately in the seriously ill patient, bretylium tosylate, procaine amide and the insertion of a temporary cardiac pacemaker to drive the heart at a fast rate.

Ventricular fibrillation (2%)

Sinus rhythm is restored with a direct current shock of 100 joules. Lignocaine is given as an intravenous bolus and continued for 2 days as a continuous infusion. Thereafter procaine amide is given, 500 mg 4 hourly for 3 weeks.

Accelerated idioventricular rhythm (20%)

Characterized by a ventricular rate of between 50–100 beats per minute. Usually benign, requiring no specific treatment.

Atrial fibrillation and atrial flutter

Digoxin 0·5 mg intravenously controls the ventricular rate. A synchronized direct current shock restoring sinus rhythm improves the cardiac output of the severely ill patient.

Bradycardia

Slow sinus rhythm due to parasympathetic reflexes will respond to intravenous atropine 0·6 mg.

Heart block (6%)

Following inferior myocardial infarction, Type I heart block is common. The right coronary artery supplies the inferior surface of the heart in 90% of people and the artery to the atrioventricular node arises from the right coronary artery at the crux of the heart.

Type I heart block is characterised by:

1 Prolonged PR interval with Wenckebach.
2 Normal shaped QRS complexes at a fairly normal rate.
3 Return to sinus rhythm after the acute episode.
4 Good prognosis, with or without temporary pacing.

Type II heart block occurs in extensive anterior myocardial infarction and is caused by interruption of the right bundle branch and interruption of the anterior and posterior divisions of the left bundle branch. Type II heart block is characterized by:

1 Practically no lengthening of the PR interval before onset of block. No Wenckebach.
2 Broad QRS complexes at a very slow rate.
3 Progression from right bundle branch block to right bundle branch block with left axis deviation and then to complete block. (The development of left axis deviation in myocardial infarction implies block of the anterior division of the left bundle branch).

Type II block requires the insertion of a pacemaker as soon as it is recognized—usually this means in the presence of right bundle branch block with left axis deviation. Rarely right axis deviation develops as a sign of block of the posterior division of the left bundle branch.

The prognosis of Type II block following myocardial infarction is poor. Even if a pacemaker is inserted, 80% die.

SHOCK

Low blood pressure, low cardiac output, low arterial oxygen tension, metabolic acidosis.

1 Continuous oxygen by face mask or in an oxygen tent only partly corrects the arterial hypoxaemia, but usually increases the blood pressure slightly.
2 Measures to increase cardiac output at present under trial are:

(i) Cautious infusion of dextrose solution, maintaining a high venous filling pressure of the heart.

(ii) Phenoxybenzamine (alpha adrenergic blocking drug). Decreases peripheral arteriolar constriction, improving tissue perfusion and possibly increasing cardiac output.

(iii) Steroids in large dosage. Produce vasodilatation.

(iv) Digoxin does not increase the cardiac output in these patients, and vasopressors are of little value because they further depress cardiac output.

HEART FAILURE

Pulmonary oedema is treated along the usual lines (p. 109).

Heart failure with evidence of salt and water retention, often appearing late in the illness, is controlled with digoxin and diuretics.

EMBOLISM

Anticoagulants may be given for the first few weeks of the illness while the patient is confined to bed, primarily for their effect in preventing thromboembolic complications. There is no proof that anticoagulants influence the short- or long-term prognosis in any other way. Anticoagulants are not used if there is generalized pericarditis, a peptic ulcer history, severe systemic hypertension, liver disease or alcoholism.

CARDIAC SURGERY IN ACUTE MYOCARDIAL INFARCTION

The initial hopes that emergency cardiac surgery in the early stages of myocardial infarction would be beneficial have not been fulfilled. Saphenous vein bypass of the occluded coronary artery with excision of any dyskinetic area of myocardium has carried a very high mortality.

Repair of a ruptured interventricular septum is often essential during the first few days because of severe failure but these emergency operations carry a high mortality and recurrence is frequent as the necrotic muscle holds stitches poorly. The prospect is good if the patient can wait 3 to 6 weeks before repair need be carried out.

Mitral regurgitation. Torrential regurgitation results when a papillary muscle becomes avulsed because its base is infarcted. Mitral valve replacement offers the only hope but few successes are recorded. Mitral regurgitation may also arise from poor function of ischaemic papillary muscles. Occasionally this is severe and requires mitral valve replacement with possibly saphenous vein bypass graft of the occluded coronary artery.

Recovery from myocardial infarction

The majority make an uncomplicated recovery and are able to return to their former occupation within 3 to 6 weeks of the infarct. Late complications include:

1 Angina pectoris—treated as described on p. 273.

2 Persistent heart failure—treated with digitalis and diuretics, having excluded a left ventricular aneurysm as the cause.

3 Sudden death from a cardiac arrhythmia—more likely if there have been severe rhythm problems during the acute phase. Long term treatment with procainamide or practolol may minimize this risk. Procainamide long term gives a high incidence of antinuclear factor in the blood and cases of systemic lupus erythematosus have **been reported.**

4 A shoulder hand syndrome—the left shoulder becomes stiff, painful and limited in movement and the left hand may also swell. This painful condition may take months to subside.

LEFT VENTRICULAR ANEURYSMS

Aetiology

Myocardial infarction

Anterior myocardial infarction (occlusion of the anterior descending artery) accounts for the vast majority of left ventricular aneurysms. Posterior infarction is a less common cause (10%). Small aneurysms can be found after 13% of cardiac infarctions but clinically significant aneurysms are much less frequent.

Aneurysm formation is more likely if an inadequate period of rest (less than 3 weeks) has followed the infarct, or if the patient has arterial hypertension. The dilated anterior wall of the left ventricle becomes replaced by fibrous tissue and clot commonly forms in it.

Other causes (rare)

Traumatic (after ventriculotomy during cardiac surgery), syphilitic, mycotic, rheumatic.

Haemodynamics

During systole the left ventricular aneurysm distends with blood and in diastole this blood returns to the left ventricular cavity. The already damaged left ventricle is performing additional useless work and may fail if the aneurysm is large.

Clinical Presentation

Symptoms

1 Previous history of myocardial infarction.

2 Left ventricular failure (dyspnoea, orthopnoea).
3 Systemic embolism (from clot in the aneurysm).

Clinical examination
Normal, except for a diffuse expansile pulsation in the region of the cardiac apex.

Electrocardiography
ST segment elevation persisting months after the infarction suggests aneurysm formation in the infarcted area.

Chest X-ray
Localized dilation on the left heart border. Serial X-rays may reveal progressive enlargement of the aneurysm. Calcification is occasionally seen in the wall of old aneurysms.

Angiography
Delineates the left ventricular cavity and shows the exact size and position of the aneurysm when the diagnosis is in doubt. Pulmonary arterial injection of the contrast is advised rather than direct left ventricular injection which may dislodge thrombus.

Prognosis

The presence of a ventricular aneurysm does not materially alter the prognosis of the original myocardial infarction. The aneurysm virtually never ruptures because the wall consists of tough fibrous tissue supported by the pericardium, and systemic embolism from contained clot is no more frequent than after infarction without aneurysm formation.

Very large aneurysms provoke left ventricular failure.

Treatment

Medical
As for the original infarct (p. 279).

Surgical

INDICATIONS FOR SURGERY
1 Large aneurysms causing left ventricular failure.
2 Recurrent embolism in spite of adequate anticoagulation.
3 Recurrent cardiac arrhythmias.

TECHNIQUE

Cardiopulmonary bypass is used, arresting the heart electrically before the aneurysm is mobilized to prevent dislodgement of clot.The aneurysm is resected and the edges of the ventricle sutured (Fig. 14.2).

If angina is a feature and narrowed arteries supplying contracting muscle have been demonstrated at angiography, saphenous vein bypass grafts are performed to those arteries. No attempt is made to revascularize the blocked artery to the aneurysm (usually the anterior descending).

The mortality of the operation is 10%, mainly from embolism at operation. Successful operation abolishes cardiac failure but the long term prognosis is governed by the extent of the patient's coronary artery disease.

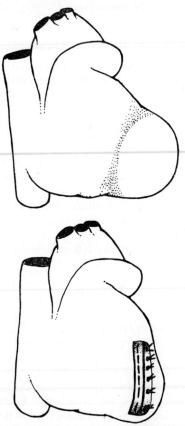

FIG. 14.2 Ventricular aneurysm and surgical excision

CHAPTER 15
SYSTEMIC HYPERTENSION AND HYPERTENSIVE HEART DISEASE

Definition of an Abnormally High Blood Pressure

No precise figures can be given for the upper limit of normal of the blood pressure because the normal range amongst the population is wide and tends to rise with age. In any one individual, also, the blood pressure varies considerably, being lowest during sleep and reaching high levels when anxious or excited. The figure of 150/90 is often suggested as the upper limit of normal, but is unsatisfactory because most of the population over the age of 55 exceed this.

There is no doubt that prolonged elevation of the blood pressure may give rise to disease and death, and in practice very high pressure readings can be taken to indicate hypertensive disease. Moderate elevation of the blood pressure is labelled hypertensive disease only when other evidence is present of the effects of prolonged hypertension such as left ventricular hypertrophy.

Physiology of the Renal-Adrenal Hormonal System

Any fall of blood pressure reducing kidney perfusion causes renin to be released from the juxta-glomerular granular cells. Renin acts enzymatically on a plasma globulin to produce angiotensin 11. Angiotensin 11 is a powerful vasopressor and also elicits aldosterone secretion. These two hormones restore renal perfusion and blood volume, thereby shutting off the initial signal for renin release.

Causes of a High Systemic Blood Pressure

Essential Hypertension (75% of all cases)
When full investigation fails to reveal an underlying cause for the high blood pressure, the hypertension is labelled *Essential Hypertension*. A family history of hypertensive disease is common, indicating that an inherited tendency to hypertension is an important factor in this group.

Renal disease (20% of all cases)
Practically any disease of the kidney can cause hypertension (release of renin is the suggested mechanism). Renal lesions causing

hypertension are bilateral in 95% of cases and the commonest are chronic pyelonephritis, chronic glomerulonephritis, polycystic disease, diabetic nephropathy, connective tissue disorders and renal artery stenosis.

Coarctation of the aorta (p. 251)

Toxaemia of pregnancy

Endocrine disease
Excessive secretion of hormones causing hypertension:
Cushing's disease: glucocorticoids.
Phaeochromocytoma: adrenaline and noradrenaline.
Conn's syndrome: aldosterone.

Collagen disease
Renal involvement is common (polyarteritis nodosa; systemic lupus erythematosus).

Drug induced
Corticosteroid medication.
Oral contraceptives increase aldosterone secretion and plasma renin, occasionally leading to the development or aggravation of hypertension.
Liquorice in amounts of 70–100 G per day causes hypertension with hypokalaemic alkalosis.
Biogastrone.

THE CLINICAL DISEASE KNOWN AS HYPERTENSIVE DISEASE

Two different diseases are described, benign and malignant hypertension, both of which have a high systemic blood pressure as their basic cause.

Benign Systemic Hypertension (98% of all cases)
Definition
A disease resulting from prolonged elevation of the arterial blood pressure but without arteriolar necrosis and without papilloedema of the optic discs.

Aetiology (p. 285)
Any of the causes of a high systemic blood pressure may be responsible.

Clinical presentation

SYMPTOMS
There are no symptoms until the onset of complications. The diagnosis is often first suggested from blood pressure readings taken at routine medical examinations.

CLINICAL EXAMINATION
1 The blood pressure is high and remains high even when there is evidence of left ventricular failure.
2 Evidence of disease produced by the hypertension includes:
   (i) Signs of left ventricular hypertrophy—heaving cardiac apex beat; fourth sound (presystolic gallop).
   (ii) Signs of arterial disease—haemorrhages and exudates in the optic fundi indicate severe disease of the arterioles. Papilloedema is absent in benign hypertension.

ELECTROCARDIOGRAM
Left ventricular hypertrophy.

CHEST X-RAY
Increase in transverse diameter of the heart, and pulmonary venous congestion when the left ventricle fails.

Investigation
1 Full investigation is necessary in every case to establish the underlying cause, particularly in patients below the age of 35 in whom essential hypertension is much less common. Special attention is given during clinical examination to:
   (i) Femoral pulses—small and delayed in coarctation of the aorta.
   (ii) Palpation of the kidneys—polycystic kidneys are palpable.
   (iii) Auscultation of the upper abdomen—fifty per cent of patients with significant renal artery stenosis have a systolic murmur. Five per cent of patients without renal artery stenosis have a systolic murmur so a murmur is not diagnostic.
2 Renal disease is confirmed or excluded by:
   (i) Examination of urine for protein, casts, red cells and bacteria.
   (ii) Blood urea.
   (iii) Intravenous pyelogram.

Chronic nephritis	Renal artery stenosis	Other structural abnormalities are usually clearly revealed
Deformed calyces and reduced renal size	Delayed appearance of contrast in pelvis of affected kidney. Increased density of contrast in later films on the affected side. Affected kidney 1·5 cm or more smaller than normal	e.g. Polycystic disease Hydronephrosis

(iv) Aortography is reserved for patients suspected to have renal artery stenosis, rather than performed routinely in every case of hypertension.

3   Endocrine diseases:

(i) Cushings disease. The diagnosis is usually obvious from clinical features of obesity, striae and hypertension. Estimation of glucocorticoid excretion confirms.

(ii) Phaeochromocytoma. Sustained hypertension or paroxysmal hypertensive attacks from excessive secretion of noradrenaline and adrenaline by tumours in the adrenal medulla or elsewhere.

Symptoms may include attacks of headache, palpitation and sweating. There is an increased incidence in patients with neurofibromatosis, Sturge Weber syndrome, tuberous sclerosis, medullary thyroid carcinoma and hyperparathyroidism.

Tumour is usually in the adrenal gland—10% are bilateral—but may be elsewhere in the abdomen including the bladder or in the thorax. Tumours are occasionally malignant.

Investigations should include measurement of 24 hour excretion of catecholamines or adrenaline metabolites such as vanilylmandelic acid in the urine as a screening test.

If positive, the excretion rates of adrenaline and noradrenaline are measured—both adrenaline and noradrenaline excess—tumour is in the adrenal gland in 95% of cases. Noradrenaline excess only—34% chance that the tumour is extra adrenal.

Location of the tumour is frequently difficult. Intravenous pyelography, aortography and peri-renal air insufflation may at times be unhelpful, leaving surgical exploration of both adrenal glands the best measure.

Treatment. Phenoxybenzamine and propranolol are given together, thereby blocking both alpha and beta actions of the catecholamines. The tumour, or tumours, may then be removed surgically.

(iii) Conn's syndrome (rare). Excessive secretion of aldosterone from an adenoma of the adrenal gland.

Symptoms may include muscular weakness, polyuria, headache, paraesthesiae and tetany. The blood pressure is only moderately elevated, retinopathy is mild and cardiac enlargement minimal.

Investigations. Serum electrolytes are the best routine screening test. Typically low serum potassium, high serum bicarbonate, high plasma volume, low haematocrit and high serum sodium concentration. Suspicion leads to estimation of plasma renin under controlled conditions of diet, posture etc. *Plasma renin is very low.*

Treatment. Spironolactone 400 mg per day restore electrolytes and blood pressure to normal. Surgical removal of an adenoma may produce complete cure.

Syndromes resembling primary aldosteronism.

Diuretic treated high blood pressure.

Hypertension with secondary aldosteronism (secondary aldosteronism is the rule in malignant hypertension). *Plasma renin excessively high, sodium low.*

Cushing's syndrome.

Liquorice induced hypertension.

4   Collagen diseases. Hypertension is rarely the presenting feature. The high erythrocyte sedimentation rate and features of systemic disease usually indicate the correct diagnosis.

Prognosis
The presence of hypertension considerably shortens the life expectancy. Death and disability occur from the complications of a high blood pressure:

CEREBRO-VASCULAR DISEASE
Much more common in hypertensive individuals than in the general population. The high blood pressure encourages the formation of aneurysms of the smaller cerebral arteries and profuse haemorrhage from a ruptured aneurysm is responsible for deaths from cerebral haemorrhage, while smaller leaks give the clinical picture of small strokes.

LEFT VENTRICULAR FAILURE
The prolonged increased load on the heart eventually exceeds the cardiac reserve.

ISCHAEMIC HEART DISEASE
Hypertension accelerates atheromatous changes in the coronary arteries.

RENAL DAMAGE

A result of the high pressure on the renal arteries.

In 'benign hypertension' the risk of developing a serious complication over a 5 year period is about 55%, reduced to 18% by effective treatment.

Treatment

INDICATIONS

Effective control of hypertension is believed to delay or prevent the onset of hypertensive complications and is indicated in:

1 Severe hypertensive disease as judged by the presence of left ventricular hypertrophy and changes in the optic fundi. The absence of symptoms does not contra-indicate treatment of this group as effective therapy reduces subsequent deaths from heart failure, cerebrovascular accidents and renal damage.

2 Hypertensive left ventricular failure. The excessive work load is removed by control of the hypertension and remarkable improvement in cardiac function results.

3 Systemic hypertension with evidence of ischaemic heart disease or cerebrovascular disease. The risk of cerebral haemorrhage is very much diminished by effective therapy. Present evidence suggests that antihypertensive therapy has little influence in the prevention of subsequent myocardial infarction.

4 Symptomless hypertension of moderate degree with no other abnormality on clinical examination. Antihypertensive therapy is advised in patients below age of 45 because of the known reduced life expectancy.

The benign nature of hypertension in some patients known to have had impressive elevations of their blood pressure for up to 30 years is well known. Recent evidence suggests that this group of patients have a low plasma renin. If confirmed, the plasma renin may be a factor in deciding which patients require therapy.

METHODS

1 SURGICAL TREATMENT of an underlying cause achieves permanent cure in a few e.g. resection of coarctation of the aorta or cure of renal artery stenosis.

2 ADEQUATE PERIODS OF SLEEP and relaxation are ensured and a sedative such as amylobarbitone (60 mg t.d.s.) is of value in the anxious, worrying individual.

3 ANTI-HYPERTENSIVE DRUGS. Effective control of the blood pressure is now possible by means of drug therapy but each drug has unpleasant, and on occasion dangerous, side effects. These drugs

control the blood pressure without affecting the cause of the hypertension and usually require to be continued indefinitely.

Beta adrenergic blocking drugs

Action Compete with catecholamines for occupation of beta-adrenergic receptor sites in the heart and elsewhere in the body. Large doses effectively lower the blood pressure without producing postural hypotension—cardiac output is reduced but the precise mode of action in hypertension is not known.

Drug Propranolol is a non-selective beta blocking drug with no intrinsic sympathomimetic activity available in tablets of 10 mgs, 40 mgs and 80 mgs. Dosage of 10 mgs four times daily is increased by increments of 25% weekly, usually requiring 400 mg/day or more for control of hypertension.

Side effects Bronchospasm from blockade of the beta receptors in the respiratory tract is troublesome in patients with a history of asthma and such patients are excluded from propranolol therapy. Heart failure—reduction of the sympathetic drive to the heart makes propranolol unsuitable for patients on the verge of cardiac failure. Bradycardia, vivid dreams, depression and claudication are not usually serious.

Place in therapy Useful in both essential and renal hypertension of all degrees of severity. Patients who respond are maintained normotensive for 24 hours a day with few side effects. This freedom makes it particularly suited to treat symptom-free young hypertensives.

Postganglionic adrenergic neurone blocking drugs

Action Blocks release of noradrenaline at the postganglionic adrenergic nerve terminals, thereby decreasing peripheral vascular resistance. Effect on the blood pressure is most marked in the standing position.

Drugs Guanethidine is long acting requiring once daily dosage. Bethanidine requires to be given four times daily. Debrisoquine is given twice or three times daily.

Side effects Postural hypotension, diarrhoea and failure of ejaculation are common. Diarrhoea is particularly associated with Guanethidine.

Place in therapy Bethanidine or Debrisoquine tablets 10 mgs are given in increasing dosage until the standing blood pressure is controlled. Very effective drugs but side effects often troublesome.

Thiazides and other oral diuretics

Action Alone these drugs produce only a slight fall in blood pressure. In combination with the more powerful drugs they potentiate the effect, allowing good control to be achieved with a lower dosage.

Drug Chlorthalidone 100 mg daily or bendrofluazide 5 mg twice daily are preferable to the more powerful diuretics, frusemide and ethacrynic acid.

Side effects Potassium loss, hyperuricaemia and gout, hyperglycaemia and diabetes.

Rauwolfia alkaloids

Action In the usual dosage e.g. reserpine 0·25 mg daily, these possess only slight hypotensive effects but they potentiate the effects of the more powerful hypotensive agents.

Side effects Nasal stuffiness, diarrhoea, gastric ulcer, muscular rigidity, and depression leading to suicide in some patients. All drugs capable of lowering the blood pressure may cause further elevation of the blood urea if severe renal damage has already occurred.

Alpha Methyldopa

Action Competes with noradrenaline for alpha receptors in blood vessels, thereby reducing vasoconstriction.

Side effects Tiredness, drowsiness, depression. Loss of effect due to tolerance. Fluid retention and oedema. Drug fever, jaundice, haemolytic anaemia.

Summary of drug therapy for hypertension

Propranolol with chlorthalidone in absence of asthma or heart failure have few side effects and often control hypertension. For quick control and where propranolol is not effective, bethanidine or debrisoquine plus chlorthalidone.

Methyldopa is less useful because of unpleasant side effects and the development of tolerance.

Malignant Hypertension (2% of all cases)

Definition

Very severe systemic hypertension, characterized clinically by the presence of papilloedema of the optic discs, and pathologically by widespread fibrinoid necrosis of arterioles.

Aetiology

Any of the causes of a high systemic blood pressure may be responsible (p. 285). Renal disease or essential hypertension is usually responsible, whereas coarctation of the aorta and hyperaldosteronism rarely cause malignant hypertension.

Peak incidence age 40–60. More common in men.

Pathology

Fibrinoid necrosis of arterioles is widespread, involving the kidneys, brain and other organs. Leakage from the damaged cerebral arterioles produces haemorrhages and exudates in the retina and oedema of the brain, while widespread involvement of renal arterioles causes progressive renal impairment. The left ventricle becomes hypertrophied from the effects of working against a high blood pressure.

Clinical presentation

SYMPTOMS

1 Cerebral and retinal involvement—headache, confusion, convulsions, coma (cerebral oedema), failing eyesight (retinopathy).

2 Left ventricular failure—dyspnoea, orthopnoea, pulmonary oedema.

3 Progressive renal impairment—anorexia, weight loss, general ill health.

CLINICAL EXAMINATION

1 The blood pressure is very high (e.g. 260/140 mm Hg).

2 Optic fundi show the results of arteriolar necrosis.

(i) Papilloedema—the intracranial pressure is high, arterial lesions having increased the fluid content of the brain.

(ii) Soft, woolly exudates—leakage of protein with fluid into the retina from damaged retinal arterioles.

(iii) Retinal haemorrhages—extravasated red blood cells from damaged arterioles.

(iv) The retinal arterioles are narrowed by spasm, a reaction to the high blood pressure.

3 Heart. Signs of left ventricular hypertrophy or failure—heaving apex beat, gallop rhythm, pulsus alternans, slight elevation of jugular venous pressure.

ELECTROCARDIOGRAM

Left ventricular hypertrophy.

CHEST X-RAY

1 Enlarged heart (left ventricular dilatation and hypertrophy).

2 Pulmonary venous congestion or frank pulmonary oedema.

RENAL FUNCTION

Progressive impairment is the rule.

1   The urine contains albumen and red cells.
2   Creatinine clearance is impaired.
3   Eventually the blood urea rises.

Investigations

As for benign hypertension (p. 287).

Prognosis

Without treatment renal failure and death usually supervene within one year. A few patients die of left ventricular failure. Effective hypotensive treatment prolongs life with remarkable regression of symptoms and signs. Failures of treatment are due to advanced renal impairment prior to the commencement of effective therapy.

	Untreated	Treated
1 year survival	20%	50–80%
5 year survival	Less than 1%	20–50

Treatment

URGENT MEASURES TO REDUCE THE BLOOD PRESSURE
1   Bed rest.
2   Potent anti-hypertensive drugs.
3   Removal of a cause for the hypertension when this is possible. Moderate reduction only of the blood pressure is attempted in cases with severe impairment of renal function because restoration of a normal blood pressure can cause further impairment.

Hypertensive Emergencies

These include acute hypertensive pulmonary oedema, hypertensive encephalopathy and malignant hypertension.
    Initial therapy is given by the parenteral route.

Drugs available

Hydrallazine 20–40 mg i.v., repeated as necessary up to a total of 500 mgs each day.
    Sodium Nitroprusside, 100 mgs in 1 litre of 5% dextrose, given very slowly i.v. using constant speed infusion pump. Duration of action is one to two minutes and almost all blood pressures can be controlled.
    Pentolinium 1–5 mgs subcutaneously increasing dose at 60 minute intervals.
    Reserpine 1–10 mgs intramuscularly, acts in 2 hours.

In the treatment of malignant hypertension oral drugs including diuretics are also given from the beginning. Salt restriction is avoided, congestive heart failure often responds without need of digitalis. Renal function is monitored during initial days of treatment.

CHAPTER 16
DISEASES OF THE PERICARDIUM

ACUTE PERICARDITIS

Definition

Acute inflammation of the pericardium, usually accompanied by a small pericardial effusion.

Aetiology

Infective

Viral (acute benign pericarditis). Coxsackie virus usually. Occasionally influenza or other viruses.

Tuberculous. Spread into the pericardium from contiguous tuberculous lymph nodes in the mediastinum.

Pyogenic. Following a streptococcal or staphylococcal septicaemia or pneumonia.

Traumatic

Recent cardiac surgery; injury to thorax.

Collagen disease

Pericarditis is a common complication of rheumatic fever, systemic lupus erythematosus, serum sickness and polyarteritis nodosa.

Neoplastic

Invasion of the pericardium by bronchogenic carcinoma or other neoplasm.

Metabolic

Pericarditis due to uraemia is a common incidental finding in renal failure.

Myocardial infarction

Local pericarditis over the infarct is present in at least 60% of patients with myocardial infarction. A generalized pericarditis complicates 15%.

Clinical Presentation

Acute benign pericarditis (Viral pericarditis)

SYMPTOMS

1 Begin with an upper respiratory tract infection in 50% of patients. General malaise, feverishness, mild perspiration and a dry cough are present at the onset of the illness, followed by the abrupt onset of pericardial pain.

2 Pericardial pain. Typically sharp and aggravated by coughing, breathing or swallowing, but may be indistinguishable from ischaemic pain. The site of the pain is usually across the chest or abdomen radiating to the shoulders and neck, but may be experienced only in the neck. The pain may persist for weeks, and recurrent attacks of pain are usual.

CLINICAL EXAMINATION

General
Fever 100–102 deg F. appears at the onset of pericarditis.

Jugular venous pressure
Becomes elevated with the development of a pericardial effusion.

Auscultation
Pericardial friction rub always present unless the pericardial effusion is large. The friction rub is a superficial scratch, usually with a *to and fro* element. The sounds are neither systolic nor diastolic, thus serving to distinguish them from cardiac murmurs. A friction rub in presystole, caused by atrial movement giving a triple cadence rub, is characteristic.

ELECTROCARDIOGRAM
ST segment elevation is usually present in many leads at the onset. Later the T waves are inverted in the leads previously showing ST elevation.

CHEST X-RAY
The transverse diameter of the heart is seen to vary on serial X-rays with the development and later regression of a pericardial effusion. A pericardial effusion cannot be differentiated from cardiac enlargement from the X-ray alone as neither the configuration of the heart shadow on the X-ray nor the change in shape with varying posture is reliable in this respect. Cardiac catheterization (a catheter along the

right border of the atrium appears well inside the cardiac shadow) and angiocardiography resolve this difficulty and are used when large chronic effusions present a problem in diagnosis.

Small bilateral pleural effusions frequently accompany a pericardial effusion (65%).

LABORATORY EVIDENCE OF ACUTE BENIGN PERICARDITIS

1   Serum glutamic oxaloacetic transaminase is elevated in less than 15% of patients and serum creatine phosphokinase is rarely elevated (differentiation from acute myocardial infarction).

2   Mild polymorphonuclear leucocytosis in the peripheral blood is usual.

3   The pericardial fluid obtained by needle pericardiocentesis is amber coloured and contains lymphocytes, but this operation is dangerous and is not required for diagnosis in the typical case.

4   The virus can be isolated from the stools, the pericardial fluid and the peripheral blood in some cases, and in others a rising antibody titre may be demonstrated in serial blood samples.

PROGNOSIS

Complications are unusual and include:

1   Cardiac tamponade (collection of fluid in the pericardial sac embarrassing the circulation by impeding the diastolic filling of the heart).

2   Cardiac arrhythmias.

3   Recurrent attacks of pain and pericarditis are common within the next 2–3 months.

4   Constrictive pericarditis is a rare sequel of viral pericarditis.

TREATMENT

1   Bed rest for the first two to three weeks usually results in prompt subsidence of symptoms. Mild analgesics are necessary for the first few days.

2   Prednisone 10 mg six hourly. Promptly relieves fever and pericardial pain of viral pericarditis but is only used in severe cases. If it is discontinued too soon, the disease recurs. Steroids do not prevent the development of large pericardial effusions.

Aspiration of pericardial fluid is necessary in the small proportion of cases where the effusion is causing cardiac tamponade. The pericardium is entered by a needle passed between the xiphisternum and the lower costal margin. Extrasystoles on the electrocardiogram during the procedure indicate that the needle point is in contact with the myocardium. Dangers of pericardiocentesis include damage to coronary vessels and intensification of tamponade by bleeding from the ventricle into the pericardium.

Features of other types of pericarditis

TUBERCULOUS

1 Few symptoms in the acute phase.
2 Pericardial fluid is often blood-stained and contains tubercle bacilli.
3 Constrictive pericarditis with calcification of the pericardium is a late sequel (p. 300) but does not occur if adequate antituberculous chemotherapy has been given early in the acute attack.

PYOGENIC

There is usually extreme toxicity.

The infecting organism can often be isolated from blood cultures and this determines the appropriate antibiotic treatment.

TRAUMATIC

Fever, general malaise, chest pain, pericardial friction rub and effusion occur within a few weeks of cardiac surgery in a small proportion of patients. This 'post-pericardiotomy syndrome' resembles acute benign pericarditis in its clinical features and prognosis.

COLLAGEN DISEASES

Rheumatic fever

Pericarditis during the acute illness indicates involvement of the heart by the rheumatic process and the incidence of chronic rheumatic valve disease is high in this group. The features of acute rheumatism (p. 126) are usually present.

Systemic lupus erythematosus

Pericarditis is occasionally the first sign of this disease. Any female patient with signs of acute pericarditis of unknown aetiology should be investigated for evidence of this disease, including a search for L.E. cells in the peripheral blood.

METABOLIC PERICARDITIS

The occurrence of pericarditis is usually a relatively unimportant incident during the course of chronic renal failure and uraemia and only occasionally results in cardiac tamponade.

PERICARDITIS IN MYOCARDIAL INFARCTION

Anticoagulants are not used when there is a generalized pericarditis because bleeding into the pericardium with cardiac tamponade may be precipitated.

CONSTRICTIVE PERICARDITIS (PICK'S DISEASE)

Definition

Gross fibrosis of the pericardium may follow various types of pericarditis, and restrict diastolic expansion of the ventricles.

Aetiology and Pathology

Tuberculosis

Tuberculous pericarditis (either blood borne or by direct invasion from a tuberculous mediastinal lymph node) used to be by far the most common cause of constrictive pericarditis until the advent of streptomycin.

The pericardium becomes grossly thickened, fibrous, calcified and even ossified, and the inflammatory process invades the underlying myocardium which becomes atrophic. The outside of the pericardium is adherent to the lung, and tuberculous pleural thickening often coexists.

Purulent and haemorrhagic pericarditis

Fibrosis and constriction occasionally ensue.

Rarer causes

Rheumatoid pericarditis, carcinomatous invasion of the pericardium, X-irradiation of the chest.

'Atypical' constrictive pericarditis

An increasingly common cause of constrictive pericarditis which occurs within a few months of non-specific (? viral) pericarditis. The pericardium is less thickened and adherent than in tuberculosis, is seldom calcified, and the underlying myocardium is neither invaded nor atrophic.

Haemodynamics

Effect on cardiac output

REDUCED CARDIAC OUTPUT

The rigid, contracted pericardium restricts diastolic filling of the ventricles and so reduces the stroke volume and the cardiac output.

BOTH VENTRICLES CONSTRICTED

The fact that both ventricles are constricted prevents the right ventricle pumping blood into the lungs which cannot be ejected by the left ventricle, as happens in left ventricular failure. The left atrial pressure does not therefore rise to high levels and dyspnoea is not a prominent symptom.

PULSUS PARADOXUS

In the normal person the blood pressure falls slightly after inspiration begins, because of the hold-up of blood in the expanding lung vessels and the fact that the increased right ventricular output has not yet reached the left ventricle. Pulsus paradoxus is an accentuation of the normal with the pulse disappearing or being markedly reduced as inspiration begins. It was called paradoxical because the pulse disappeared without there being any change in the apical cardiac impulse.

The mechanism is probably that the normal increased filling of the right ventricle on inspiration shifts the septum and further compresses the left ventricle within the constricted pericardial cavity. Also the pulmonary venous pressure drops on inspiration but the left atrial pressure does not. This reversed pressure gradient reduces the blood flow from pulmonary veins to left atrium and the stroke volume falls.

Effect on venous pressures

BOTH LEFT AND RIGHT ATRIAL PRESSURES ARE
EQUALLY RAISED

During diastole blood fills all four chambers of the heart until expansion is terminated by the rigid pericardium.

KUSSMAUL'S SIGN

In the normal person the jugular venous pressure falls during inspiration because the intrathoracic pressure falls—blood flow into the thorax increases and right ventricular output rises to accommodate it.

In constrictive pericarditis the jugular venous pressure may rise on inspiration, probably because the constricted right ventricle is unable to accept the increased systemic venous return.

Y DESCENT AND TROUGH (FRIEDREICH'S SIGN)

In classical constrictive pericarditis the dominant wave in the jugular venous pulse is a *y* descent. As the tricuspid valve opens, blood flows rapidly into the right ventricle and the raised venous pressure drops sharply, only to rise again when filling ceases as the ventricle is brought up against the rigid pericardium.

SYSTOLIC DESCENT

Less frequently in constrictive pericarditis the dominant wave is a systolic rather than a diastolic descent. The myocardium is normal in these patients and not atrophic and invaded as it is by tuberculous pericarditis. The explanation of the dominant systolic descent is that the cardiac output is efficiently and quickly ejected, which temporarily lowers the volume of blood in the pericardial box allowing blood to flow into the heart during systole. If this volume change can be transferred to the atria (fluid or soft pericardial constriction), the jugular venous pressure falls during systole.

Effect on auscultatory signs

THIRD SOUND

In classical constrictive pericarditis there is an early high-pitched 3rd sound falling 0·1 sec after aortic valve closure. Expansion of the ventricles is terminated sooner than usual by the constricted pericardium, and the A–V valves are vibrated by the shock to produce an early third sound.

Clinical Presentation of Classical Constrictive Pericarditis (Pick's Disease)

Symptoms

1   Previous history of tuberculosis or pericarditis is unusual.
2   Onset of symptoms is insidious.
3   Dyspnoea is slight (left atrial pressure only moderately raised).
4   Fatigue (low cardiac output).
5   Oedema and ascites are the main symptoms (raised systemic venous pressure).

Clinical examination

PULSE AND BLOOD PRESSURE

Pulse small (reduced pulse pressure and cardiac output) and sometimes paradoxical, almost disappearing during inspiration (increased right ventricular filling compressing left ventricle). Low blood pressure.

JUGULAR VENOUS PRESSURE

Raised and sometimes rising further on inspiration—Kussmaul sign (right ventricle unable to accept increased flow into thorax). Dominant wave is *y* descent and trough (abrupt relaxation of atrophic right ventricle as tricuspid valve opens).

CARDIAC IMPULSES
Barely palpable (fibrosis around ventricles). Systolic retraction of the apex is characteristic when the apex beat is palpable.

AUSCULTATION
Early third sound (rapid ventricular filling abruptly halted).

ENLARGED LIVER, ASCITES AND OEDEMA
(Raised systemic venous pressure.)

Electrocardiography
Widespread T inversion (chronic pericarditis). Atrial fibrillation in one-third of patients.

Chest X-ray
Heart size normal or slightly enlarged (thick pericardium). Calcification in pericardium is usual, but not invariable.

Cardiac catheterization
Simultaneous right and left atrial pressures are both raised equally at rest and rise together on exercise (both ventricles equally constricted).

Distinction from Cardiomyopathy

1 Dyspnoea is marked in cardiomyopathy (high left atrial pressure).
2 Heart size is larger (failing ventricle).
3 The left atrial pressure rises significantly higher than the right on exercise (right ventricular function better than left).

Clinical Presentation of Atypical (post-viral) Constrictive Pericarditis

As classical Pick's Disease but:
1 Arises relatively soon after viral pericarditis.
2 Dominant *systolic* descent in jugular venous pressure (right atrium fills when blood is ejected from rigid cavity. Different from Pick's disease because A–V ring can move down and allow right atrial filling).
3 No third sound (good myocardium).
4 Often no calcium.

5   Operation simpler than Pick's disease (myocardium not so invaded by calcium) and postoperative course smoother (good myocardium).

Treatment

Only surgical removal of the thickened pericardium is of curative value.

Indications for surgery
The presence of oedema and ascites.

Technique
Bilateral 4th intercostal space, left thoracotomy or median sternotomy incision, mobilization and removal of pericardium from ventricles and A–V groove. Antituberculous cover is not usually necessary as the tuberculous process is no longer active.

Results

MORTALITY 15%
From technical difficulty (calcium and bone invading myocardium) and post-operative cardiac failure and respiratory complications (myocardium affected by disease).

POST-OPERATIVE FUNCTION
Higher than normal venous pressure and third sound may persist if the myocardium is badly involved, but symptoms disappear.

RECONSTRICTION
5–10% (usually due to inadequate first operation).

CARDIAC TRAUMA AND TAMPONADE

Types of Cardiac Trauma

Blunt chest injury
Deceleration injuries (car and aeroplane accidents), acceleration injuries (pedestrians struck by cars), crush injuries (e.g. weight falling on chest).

Penetrating chest injury
Stabbing, gunshot wounds, cardiac surgery.

Other causes
Perforation by cardiac catheter.

Effects of Trauma

Damage to functional components of the heart
1 Myocardium—myocardial contusions and lacerations and damage to coronary arteries may lead to infarction.
2 Ventricular septum—perforation produces a ventricular septal defect.
3 Valves—rupture of valve cusps or papillary muscles may be caused by either blunt or penetrating injury.
4 Conduction mechanism—heart block and other arrhythmias result.

Lacerations within the pericardium causing tamponade
Lacerations of ventricles, atria or great vessels allow rapid haemorrhage into the pericardial sac.

Aortic lacerations outside the pericardium
Aortic lacerations are due to blunt or penetrating injury and may be closed by clot, allowing the patient to reach hospital (p. 258).

Cardiac tamponade
Compression of the heart by fluid in the pericardium, which may be blood (trauma, ruptured aneurysms) or inflammatory exudate (any pericarditis).

HAEMODYNAMICS OF TAMPONADE

Poor ventricular filling
The presence of fluid in the pericardium prevents adequate filling of the ventricles during diastole. The jugular venous pressure rises, the blood pressure falls and a reflex tachycardia occurs. Death ensues when the intrapericardial pressure reaches about 17 cms of water which may occur with as little as 200 ml acutely. In more chronic cases there is time for dilatation of the pericardium allowing large effusions to form.

Systolic descent in jugular venous pressure (p. 303)

Pulsus paradoxus
The pulse pressure markedly diminishes during inspiration (p. 12).

Clinical Presentation of Patient with Recent Cardiac Trauma

Symptoms
History of recent injury.

Clinical examination

GENERAL

Evidence of a blunt or penetrating chest injury is usually but not always obtained.

SIGNS OF HAEMORRHAGE (if the heart is lacerated)

Pallor, sweating, tachycardia, hypotension, low jugular venous pressure.

SIGNS OF TAMPONADE (when bleeding is into pericardium)

Tachycardia, pulsus paradoxus, hypotension, raised jugular venous pressure with a systolic descent, diminished heart sounds. The diagnosis of tamponade is confirmed by pericardial aspiration.

ARRHYTHMIAS

Atrial fibrillation, heart block, ventricular extrasystoles and fibrillation can all result from cardiac injury.

MURMURS OF TRAUMATIC VALVE INCOMPETENCE AND SEPTAL DEFECTS (rare)

Electrocardiography
High peaked T waves may indicate blood in the pericardium. Changes of myocardial ischaemia and infarction may be seen. Arrhythmias are frequent. A triad virtually diagnostic of pericardial effusion is low voltage, ST segment elevation and electrical alternans.

Chest X-ray
Widening mediastinum on serial films indicates a ruptured aorta or dissecting aneurysm. Haemothorax and fractured ribs are common.

Prognosis

Sixty to seventy per cent of patients with penetrating injuries of the heart die before reaching hospital, but up to 85% of the remainder can be rescued by efficient treatment.

Treatment

Conservative management
Treatment is initially conservative.

MYOCARDIAL CONTUSION
As for myocardial infarction (rest, sedation, etc.) except that anti-coagulants are contra-indicated.

LACERATIONS INSIDE THE PERICARDIUM
Tamponade is corrected by pericardial aspiration with a wide bore needle inserted beside the xiphoid process, accompanied by transfusion to replace blood loss.

Surgery

INDICATIONS FOR OPERATION
1   Persistence or recurrence of signs of tamponade after one pericardial aspiration. The blood in the pericardium is often clotted (the rapid rate of bleeding prevents the defibrinating action of the beating heart) and then cannot be withdrawn through a needle.
2   Increasing widening of the mediastinum or enlarging haemothorax on serial chest X-rays.

TECHNIQUE
Left anterior thoracotomy and suture of lacerations.

Results of treatment

CARDIAC LACERATIONS
Conservative management by aspiration has surprisingly been shown to have a better survival rate (up to 85% of those reaching hospital alive) than surgery, but necessarily such a series includes mainly the smaller wounds. Best results are obtained if immediate surgery is available when a single, or at the most two, pericardial aspirations fail to resuscitate the patient.

AORTIC LACERATIONS
Thirty per cent of those reaching hospital alive may survive if immediate thoracotomy and suture of the lacerations are performed.

CHAPTER 17
COR PULMONALE

Definition

Hypertrophy of the right ventricle resulting from disease affecting primarily the structure or function of the lung.

The pulmonary arterial disease caused by congenital or acquired heart disease is not usually included under the term 'cor pulmonale'.

Aetiology

Right ventricular hypertrophy is a result of increased resistance to pulmonary blood flow. The increased resistance may be due to constriction of the pulmonary arterioles, organic narrowing, or a reduction of the total pulmonary vascular bed. Lung diseases responsible for these changes are:

1 Diseases affecting the alveoli or the air passages of the lung—chronic bronchitis with generalized airway obstruction, with or without emphysema; bronchial asthma; primary emphysema; pulmonary fibrosis due to tuberculosis, pneumoconiosis, bronchiectasis, radiation, sarcoidosis, chronic diffuse interstitial fibrosis.

2 Diseases primarily affecting the movements of the thoracic cage —kyphoscoliosis; chronic neuromuscular weakness (poliomyelitis, obesity with alveolar hypoventilation).

3 Diseases primarily affecting the pulmonary vasculature—multiple pulmonary emboli (p. 86); primary pulmonary hypertension (p. 84); primary pulmonary thrombosis.

Haemodynamics

In all cases of cor pulmonale the resistance to blood flow through the lungs is high, although there is a wide variation in pulmonary artery pressure from case to case. Right ventricular hypertrophy is a result of the increased work of maintaining the pulmonary blood flow.

Clinical Presentation of Cor Pulmonale Secondary to Chronic Bronchitis and Emphysema

Symptoms

1 Early—cough and expectoration for many years, present particularly in the winter.

2 Intermediate—progressively disabling acute respiratory infections accompanied by dyspnoea and wheeze.

3 Late—dyspnoea on slight exertion with peripheral oedema and central cyanosis. Symptoms become much worse during any exacerbation of the bronchitis due to respiratory failure, when mental confusion or coma may appear.

Clinical examination

GENERAL

Laboured breathing employing the accessory muscles of respiration (obstructive airway disease).

Central cyanosis (underventilated alveoli fail to oxygenate the blood passing through them).

Mental confusion or disorientation (raised Pco_2 and hypoxia).

Warm peripheral extremities (peripheral vasodilatation and cardiac output at upper limit of normal, due to anoxia and high Pco_2).

Peripheral oedema (salt and water retention due in part to right ventricular failure).

JUGULAR VENOUS PRESSURE

Elevated when there is salt and water retention and right ventricular failure.

PRECORDIAL PALPATION

Overlying lung disease usually obscures any evidence of right ventricular hypertrophy.

AUSCULTATION

Heart sounds faint (poor transmission of heart sounds through the lungs). Loud pulmonary valve closure sound (high pulmonary artery pressure). Third heart sound arising from the right ventricle (right ventricular failure).

LUNGS

Limited expiratory excursion; hyper-resonance to percussion (overinflated lungs); faint breath sounds, wheezing and prolonged expiration (expiration in particular is obstructed by bronchiolar collapse).

Electrocardiography

1 Frequently normal despite the presence of right ventricular hypertrophy (right ventricular hypertrophy is not gross in cor pulmonale and the transmission of electrical activity in the heart to the body surface is considerably disturbed by the presence of the diseased lungs).

2 A proportion of cases fulfil the electrocardiographic criteria for the diagnosis of right ventricular hypertrophy (see p. 45).

Chest X-ray

1 Evidence of emphysema—localized areas of transradiancy in the lung fields suggesting bullae. Vascular shadows in the peripheral lung fields sparse and widely spaced. Low flat diaphragm lying below the level of the 7th rib anteriorly.

2 Dilatation of the main pulmonary artery and its large branches (pulmonary hypertension).

3 The heart shadow is often small, because of the low diaphragm. When failure occurs the heart shadow is increased in size.

Respiratory function tests

1 Forced vital capacity is reduced (high residual volume).

2 Forced expiratory volume during the first second (F.E.V.1.) is reduced considerably below the normal i.e. below 75% of the forced vital capacity (expiration obstructed by narrowing of the bronchioles).

3 Oxygen tension and saturation of the arterial blood are reduced and the carbon dioxide tension increased (failure of the lungs to perform respiration efficiently).

Treatment

Prevention of chronic bronchitis

Cigarette smoking plays a large part in the production of chronic bronchitis. Other less important factors include atmospheric pollution, working in an overcrowded or dusty environment and severe respiratory tract infections. Some measure of control is possible for all four factors, particularly cigarette smoking.

Treatment of chronic bronchitis and cor pulmonale

GENERAL

Severe complications and complete disability may be postponed or prevented if cigarette smoking is permanently discontinued, a dust-free working environment ensured and acute respiratory tract infections promptly treated with antibiotics, such as tetracycline 250 mg q.d.s. for 10 days.

TREATMENT OF AN ACUTE EXACERBATION OF BRONCHITIS

1 Antibiotics in full dosage, the choice depending on the infecting organism. Haemophilus influenzae is usually the cause of the exacerbation and tetracycline or ampicillin may prove the most effective antibiotics.

2 Oxygen by special Venturi face mask. This effectively raises the level of oxygen in the inspired air and is unlikely to cause a build up of CO_2.

3 Respiratory stimulants. Some bronchodilatation and consequent improvement in ventilation can usually be achieved by drugs such as intravenous aminophylline, or isoprenaline or ephedrine by mouth.

4 Tracheostomy and artificial ventilation. This may be necessary to tide the patient over a period of acute respiratory failure.

Morphine, and practically every other type of sedative, are respiratory depressants and will further aggravate respiratory insufficiency.

TREATMENT OF HEART FAILURE

Heart failure first appears during an episode of acute respiratory infection. Treatment of the infection, thereby re-establishing adequate oxygenation of the lungs, is most important as this will produce a substantial drop in the pulmonary artery pressure. Digitalis and other diuretics are given in addition to the above measures when peripheral oedema appears.

CHAPTER 18

CARDIOMYOPATHY

Definition

Primary myocardial disease. Cardiac diseases in which the fault lies within the myocardium.

Disorders of the heart due to rheumatic, hypertensive, coronary artery disease, congenital cardiac lesions or thyroid disease are excluded.

Aetiology

1 *Idiopathic*: the provoking cause cannot be identified in the large majority of patients.

2 *Familial*: occurring in several members of a family, usually this is of the hypertrophic or the hypertrophic obstructive type.

3 *Toxic*: emetine, arsenic, cobalt, ethylene glycol have all been identified as toxic to the myocardium.

Alcohol plays an important part in many patients but it is not known if this is a direct toxic effect.

4 *In neuromyopathic diseases*: Friedreich's ataxia; progressive muscular dystrophy; myotonic muscular dystrophy.

5 *Infiltrative*: Haemochromatosis—deposition of iron; glycogen storage diseases; gargoylism—infiltration with cells containing mucopolysaccharides; amyloidosis, sarcoidosis, scleroderma, systemic lupus erythematosus.

6 *Postpartum*: (occurring during the second to the twentieth week postpartum—cause unknown), nutritional deficiency (beriberi).

7 *Myocarditis*: from Coxsackie B virus, influenza, infectious mononucleosis, diphtheria, Chaga's disease have been recognized. It may be that these agents produce a chronic cardiomyopathy long after the acute recognizable infection is over but this is unproven in man.

Pathology

The left ventricle is practically always involved, and often the right ventricle is also affected. Four types are described:

1 *Hypertrophic*—generalized hypertrophy of the left ventricle.
2 *Hypertrophic with left ventricular outflow obstruction*—p. 157.
3 *Congestive*—dilated chambers with cardiac failure.

4 *Restrictive*—filling is restricted, giving the features of constrictive pericarditis.

The usual findings are cardiac enlargement and hypertrophy, absence of significant coronary luminal narrowing, dilatation and hypertrophy of all chambers and, microscopically, myocardial fibre hypertrophy with minimal inflammatory reaction. Mural thrombi are present in over 20%.

Pathologically distinct types are:

1 Endomyocardial fibrosis. Common in West Africa, the typical features being fibrosis of the endocardium involving the papillary muscles and chordae of the mitral and tricuspid valves.
2 Fibro-elastosis. Thickening of the endocardium of infants and children in association with cardiac failure. Severe congenital cardiac defects or valve lesions are usually present in this group.

Clinical Presentation of Cardiomyopathy

There are three modes of presentation.
1 Unexplained cardiomegaly, possibly without symptoms.
May be family history of sudden death before age 50.
2 Congestive heart failure in the absence of an identifiable cause. Gallop rhythm is a constant finding, a third or fourth heart sound from left or right ventricle or from both ventricles.
Atrioventricular valve regurgitation is common, giving a pansystolic murmur when the left or right ventricle is dilated, the murmur vanishing with treatment of heart failure.
History of alcoholism or other toxic cause may be obtained in some.
3 Symptoms and some signs of aortic stenosis (hypertrophic obstructive cardiomyopathy).
A sharp rising arterial pulse is one of the main differentiating features, see p. 157.

Occasionally cardiomyopathy may present as an unexplained cardiac tachyarrhythmia or heart block, or closely mimic the clinical features of constrictive pericarditis (cardiac amyloidosis is the classic example of this).

Diagnosis of Cardiomyopathy

A family history of unusual heart disease may be obtained, particularly in hypertrophic obstructive cardiomyopathy. Gallop rhythms are very common and the absence of a clear gallop rhythm in congestive heart failure is a point against the diagnosis. The electrocardiogram is usually abnormal, with one or more of the following features:

1   Left atrial enlargement.
2   Left ventricular hypertrophy.
3   Multifocal ventricular extrasystoles, atrial fibrillation, ventricular tachycardia, conduction disturbances both atrioventricular and intraventricular.

Chest X-ray: cardiomegaly with fluctuations in heart size, returning to near normal after treatment early in the course of the congestive cardiomyopathies is the rule. Pulmonary venous congestion often seen due to left ventricular failure.

Prognosis

Acute primary myocardial disease may disappear with no residual damage or may perhaps present years later as idiopathic cardiomyopathy, although this has yet to be firmly proved in man. Alternatively, acute cardiomyopathies may present as dangerous arrhythmias or as progressive heart failure ending in death.

Chronic cardiomyopathy may remain stable for years but ultimately progresses slowly or rapidly to congestive failure. Sudden death from cardiac arrhythmia and pulmonary or systemic embolism can appear at any stage.

Treatment

In the few cases where a cause is identified appropriate action is taken.

Alcohol is forbidden in any case where the consumption is high, whether alcohol is believed to be the major cause or not. A high protein diet is ensured. Systemic diseases such as hyperthyroidism or anaemia are controlled as these may be contributory to the condition.

Occupations or sports involving sustained physical exertion should be avoided.

Bed rest for several weeks at the onset of each episode of congestive heart failure is clearly beneficial. Prolonged bed rest for a year or more is impracticable and the reported benefit has not been unequivocably established.

Digitalization and diuretic therapy is used to control cardiac failure. Care is necessary because overdigitalization is possible, either because of increased myocardial sensitivity or because large dosage is used in a vain effort to control an intractable arrhythmia.

Pacemaker insertion is required when dealing with arrhythmias causing syncope or when large dosages of antiarrhythmic drugs are used.

Anticoagulants are indicated if there is evidence of pulmonary or systemic embolism or for congestive failure with atrial fibrillation where the risk of embolism is high. Restoration of sinus rhythm by direct current shock can dramatically improve some patients. Anticoagulants are advised prior to this procedure.

CHAPTER 19
TUMOURS OF THE HEART

Pathology

Secondary deposits in the myocardium and pericardium

Metastases from malignant disease elsewhere are twelve times as common as primary tumours of the heart but are seldom of clinical significance, being found as incidental findings at post-mortem.

Primary intracardiac tumours

MYOXMA (50% of all primary tumours)

A polypoid mass of gelatinous tissue usually in the left atrium (75%), attached by a pedicle to the fossa ovalis, atrial appendage or origin of a pulmonary vein. The right atrium is a less common site. It consists of myxomatous tissue with scanty blood vessels and small haemorrhages.

A myxoma is benign but may recur if it is not totally removed. Its presence causes illness and death because of prolapse into the mitral valve, and because fragments break off as systemic or pulmonary emboli.

SARCOMA (20% of primary tumours)

All types of sarcoma occur, usually in the right atrium, and death occurs rapidly from extension through the wall of the heart into the pericardium rather than from proliferation into the chambers like a myxoma.

OTHER TUMOURS

Fibroma, rhabdomyoma, lipoma, angioma etc. are rare

Clinical Presentation of Left Atrial Myxoma

Types of presentation

Left atrial myxoma may present in three ways:

1 Symptoms and signs of mitral valve obstruction. Tumour prolapsing into valve.
2 Systemic embolism. Friable fragments of tumour.
3 Generalized toxaemia. The cause of this is unknown.

Distinction from mitral stenosis

1 Signs of severe pulmonary hypertension (jugular venous a wave, right ventricular hypertrophy, loud pulmonary second sound and pulmonary venous hypertension on chest X-ray out of proportion to the minimal mitral stenotic signs. Due to mitral valve obstruction being in fact severe and to the piston effect of the large v wave as the tumour is expelled back into the left atrium.

2 Wide splitting of 1st heart sound. T_1 is audible because of pulmonary hypertension and M_1 is delayed because it takes time for the tumour to be ejected into the atrium and the mitral valve to close.

3 Pansystolic murmur. Mild mitral regurgitation with the tumour in the valve.

4 'Tumour thud'. Tumour falling back into ventricle. Thud has timing of opening snap (i.e. 0·1 sec or less after A_2) but is a dull sound.

5 Variable mid diastolic murmur. Usually soft and may be altered by posture.

6 Signs of general toxaemia. Weight loss, finger clubbing, anaemia, splenomegaly, raised ESR and altered plasma proteins.

7 Echocardiography. Thin line of normal anterior leaf of mitral valve is shown with large echo from tumour behind.

8 Cardiac catheterization. High pulmonary artery pressure. Large v wave on indirect LA (wedge) pressure with steep 'y' descent.

9 Angiography. Contrast is injected into the pulmonary artery rather than left atrium to avoid dislodging friable tumour fragments. A filling defect is usually, though not always, seen.

Distinction from mitral stenosis may be difficult. Angiography and echocardiography are the most reliable methods.

Clinical Presentation of Right Atrial Myxoma

Presents as tricuspid stenosis or insufficiency (fatigue, raised jugular venous pressure, enlarged liver, serous effusions and oedema, with a P pulmonale on electrocardiography and enlarged right atrium on chest X-ray).

Cardiac catheterization reveals a diastolic gradient across the tricuspid valve and angiography shows a filling defect in the atrium.

Clinical Presentation of Sarcoma

Presents as malignant pericardial disease (retrosternal pain, tachycardia, pulsus paradoxus, raised jugular venous pressure, enlarged heart shadow) with death being due to tamponade or cardiac rupture. The diagnosis is made by aspiration of a blood-stained pericardial effusion containing malignant cells.

Treatment

Myxoma (and other benign tumours)
Surgical treatment is urgent because fatal embolism or total obstruction of the mitral valve may suddenly occur. With cardiopulmonary bypass and an arrested heart to prevent embolism from the fragile tumour, the atrium is opened, the myxoma removed and its base excised to prevent recurrence.

Sarcoma
No effective treatment is available.

INDEX